Thérèse Dufour and Marie-Claire Hamon
Illustrations by Thanh Portal
Translated by Dipa Chaudhuri

Clever like a monkey

Adapted from a traditional African tale

A tale along with postures for being joyful

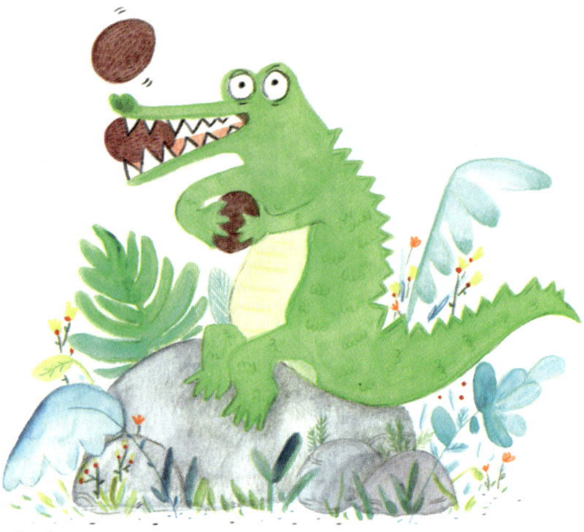

Om Books International

Open yourself up to joy

To start with, open yourself up to joy.

Benefit: This posture connects the child to an inner state of joy.

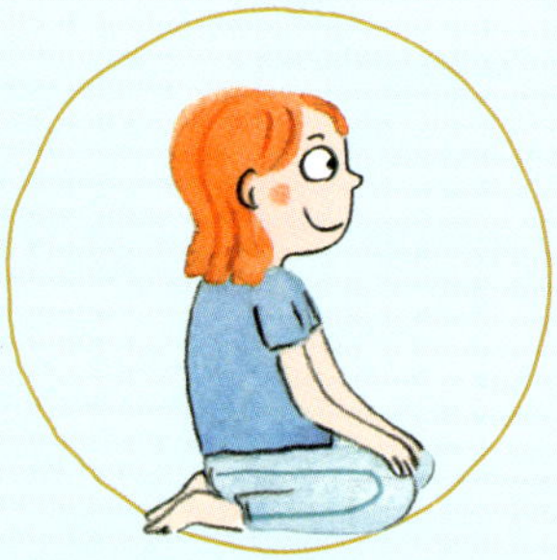

Sit down on your heels and place your hands on your thighs.

4 breaths

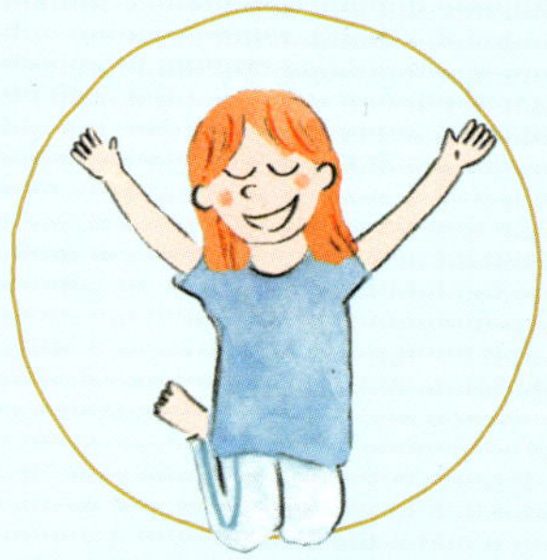

Open your hands, chest, and the palms of your hands wide. You are opening yourself up to joy.

4 breaths

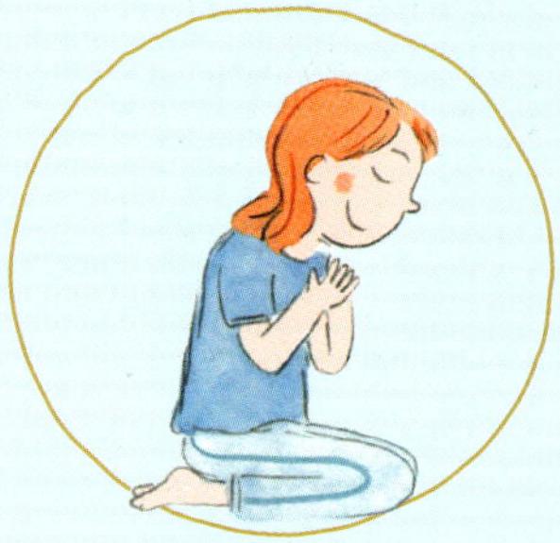

Join your hands in front of your heart and bow your head.

In a beautiful African forest, in the midst of a river flowing through it, is an island.

This island is a veritable paradise: out here, one can eat delicious seeds and leaves, crunchy insects, fleshy and fragrant coconuts, just about the best in the world!

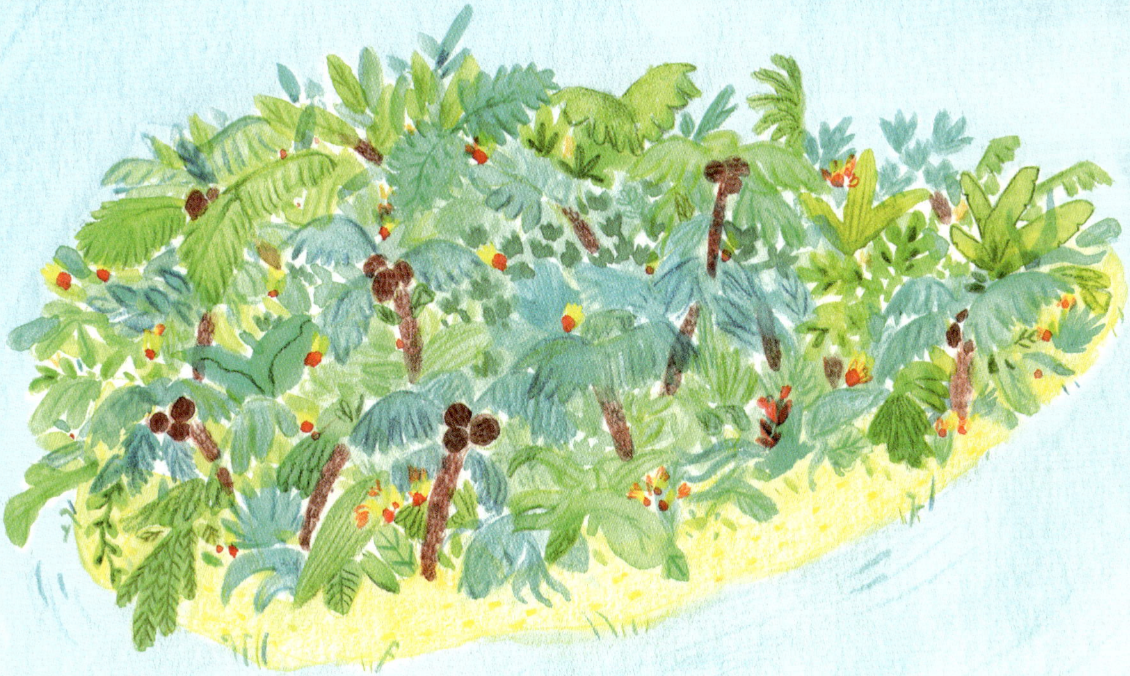

Malisco, the small monkey, would love to go there, but he doesn't know how to swim... And Denduratou, the old crocodile who would love to make a good meal of him, keeps an eye on his goings and comings every time the little monkey ventures close to the river.

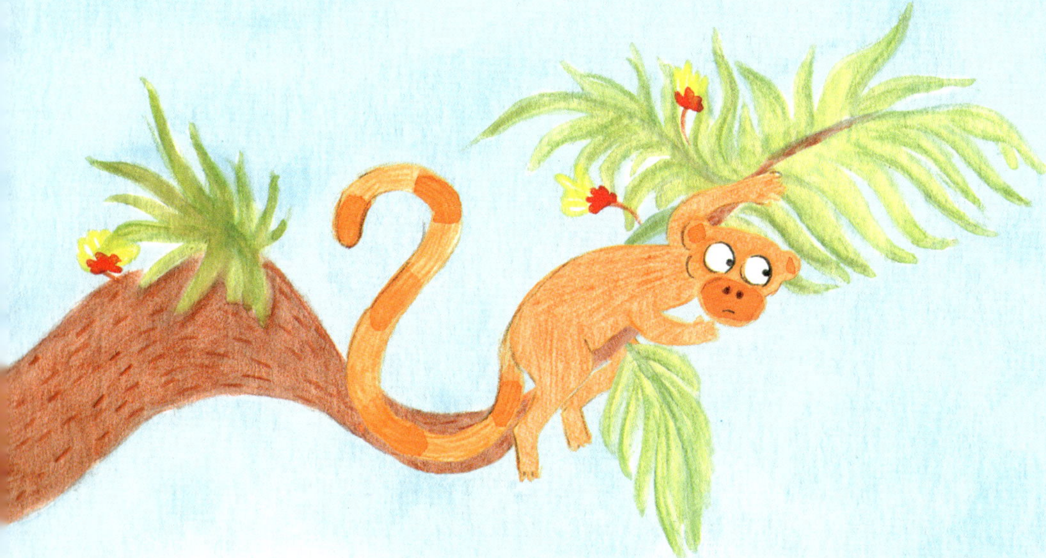

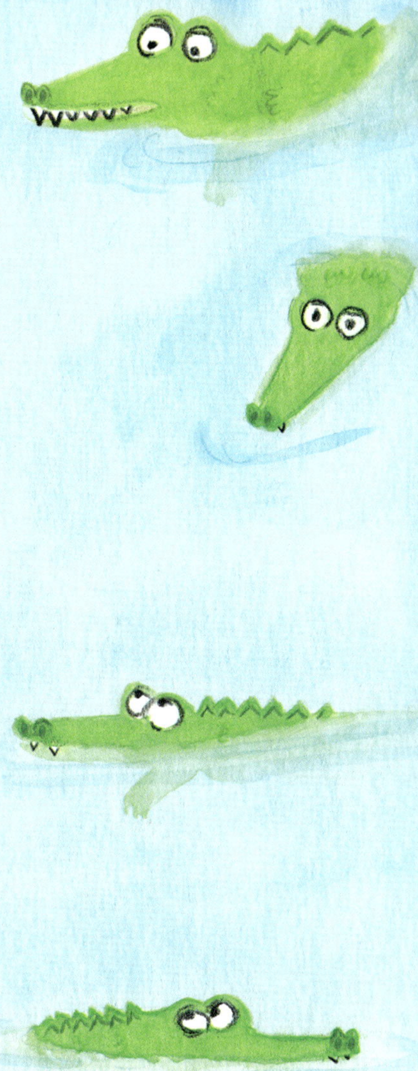

The crocodile

You are a crocodile and a hungry one at that!

Benefit: This posture tones up the back and shoulder muscles.

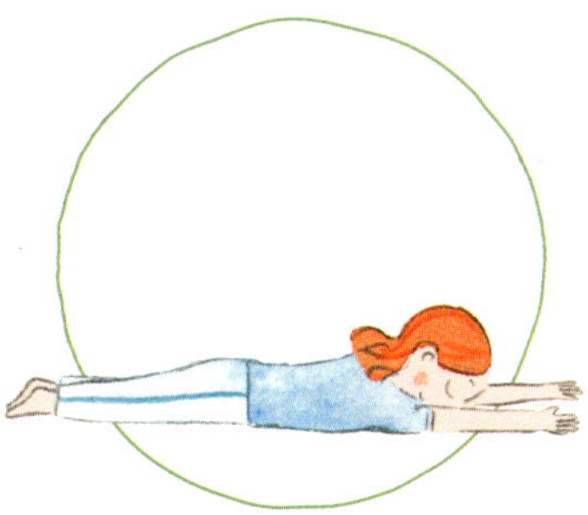

Lie down on your stomach and stretch your hands in front of yourself.

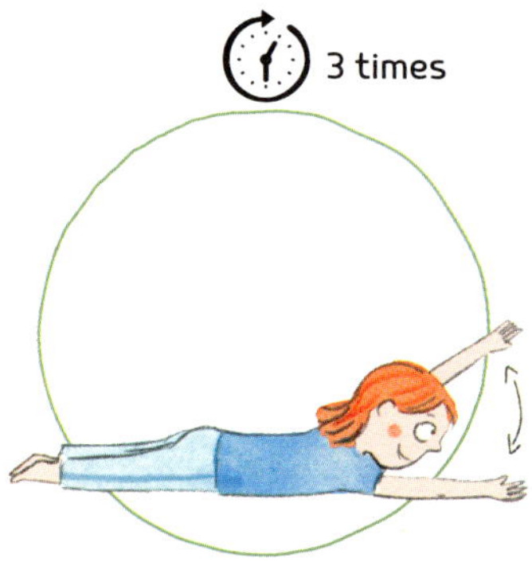

Lift your face from the ground. Lift and bring down one of the outstretched hands. Open and close Denduratou's jaws.

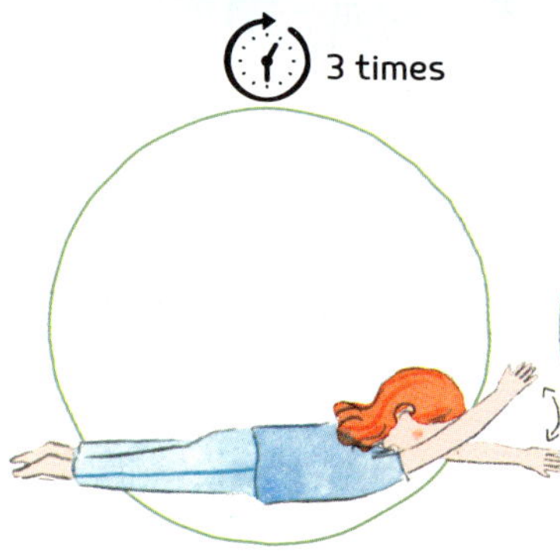

Do the same thing with the other hand.

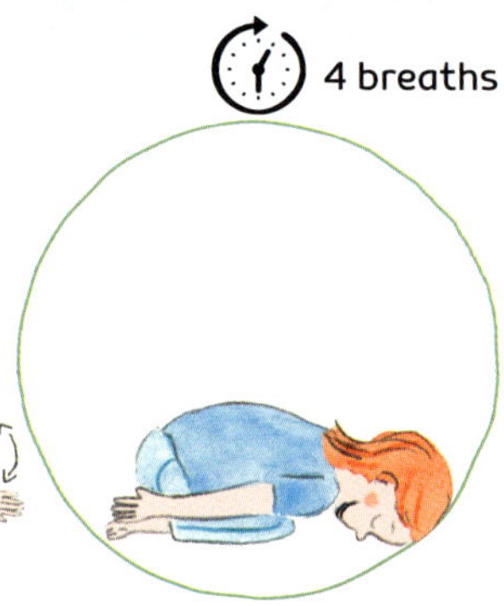

Sit down on your heels and touch the forehead to the ground, with your hands by the side of your body.

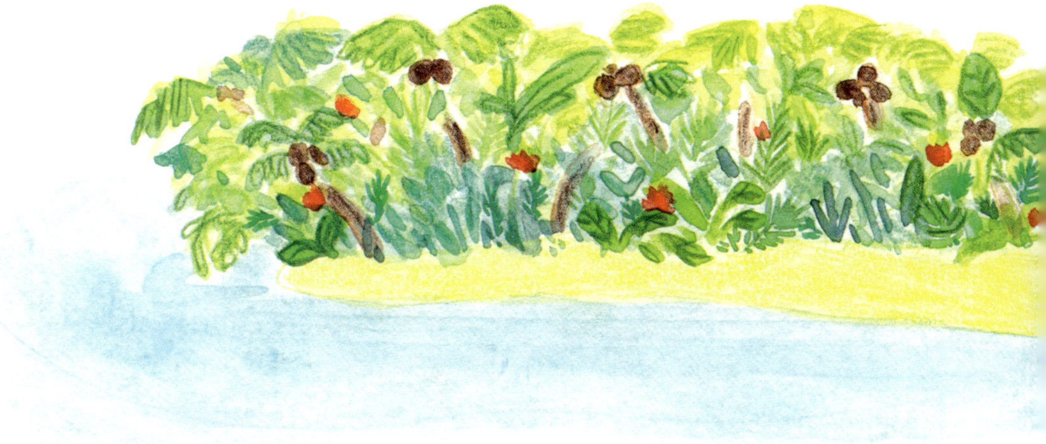

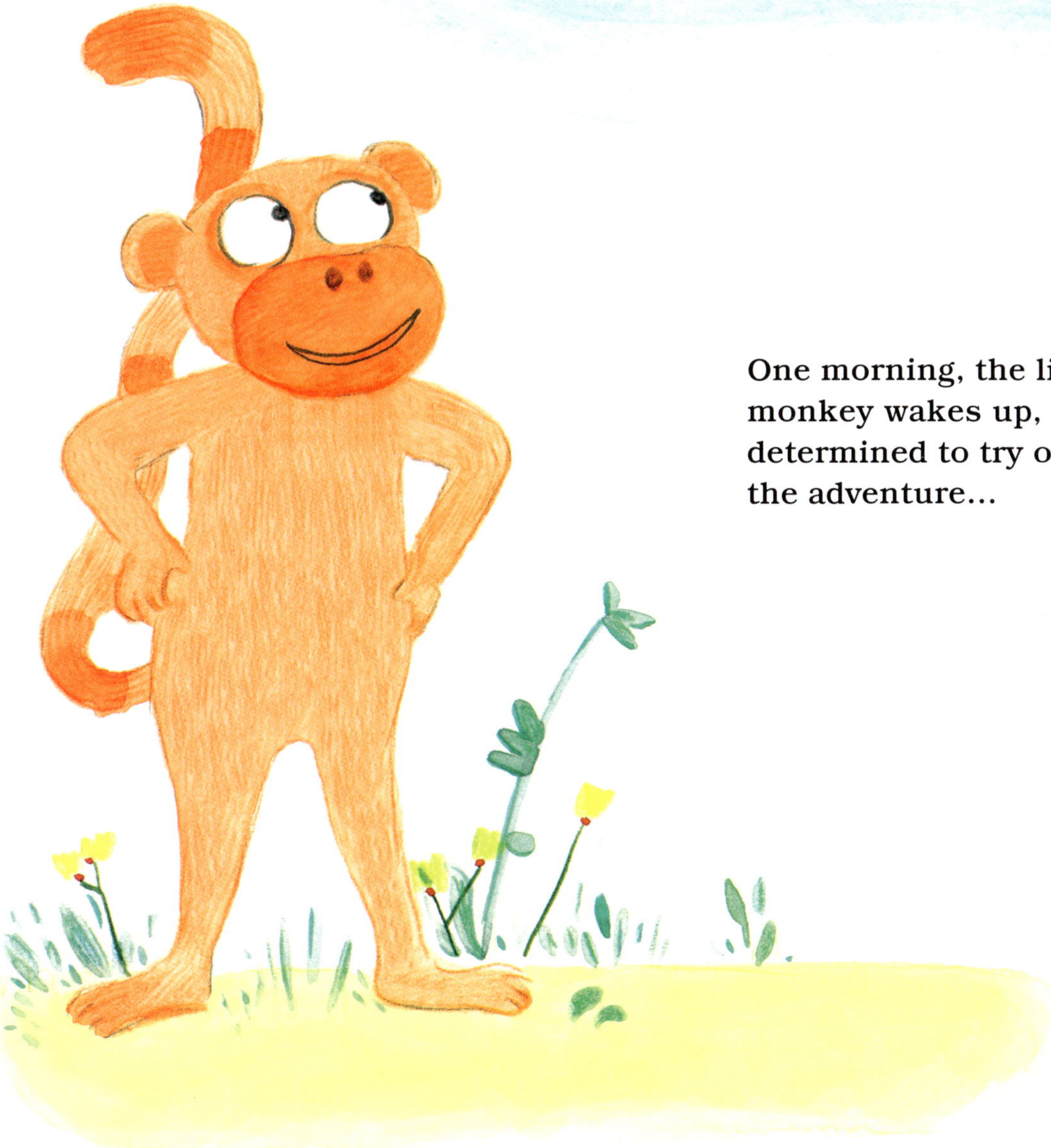

One morning, the little monkey wakes up, determined to try out the adventure...

Close to the river, on a large stretch of land, pink flamingos rest before resuming their route.

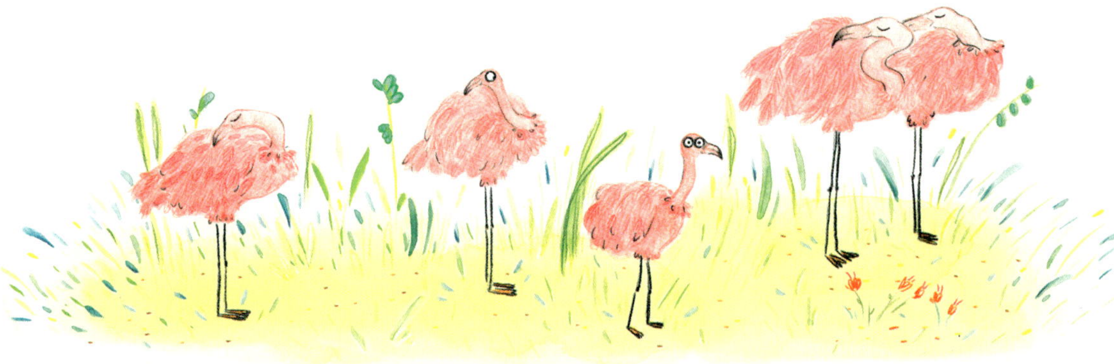

Malisco speaks to Long Legs, the chief: "If you agree to transport me to the island, I shall show you a hiding place full of exquisite insects."
"Fine," replies the chief.

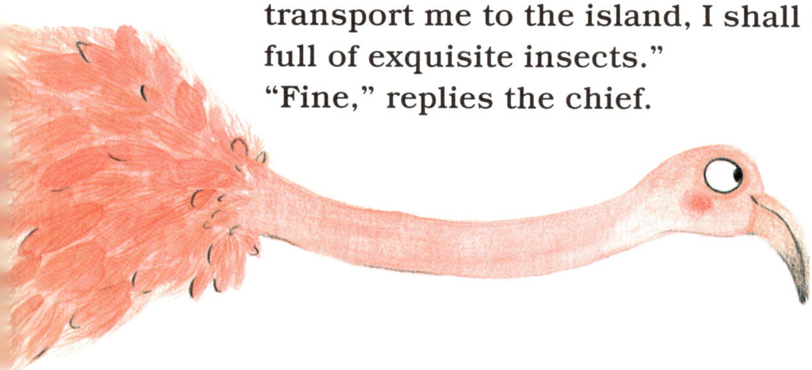

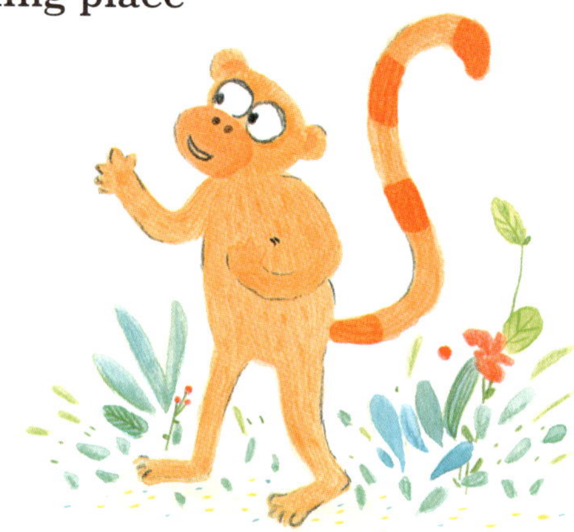

The flight of the pink flamingo

Like the bird, take flight! To help maintain your balance, open your eyes wide.

Benefit: This posture associates balance with movement.

4 breaths

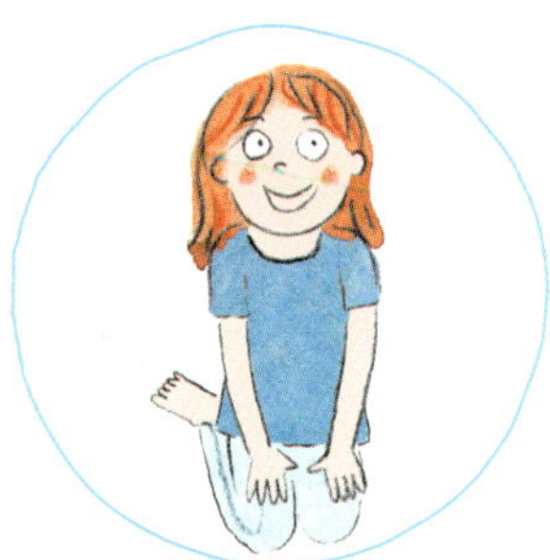

Get down on your knees and sit on your heels.

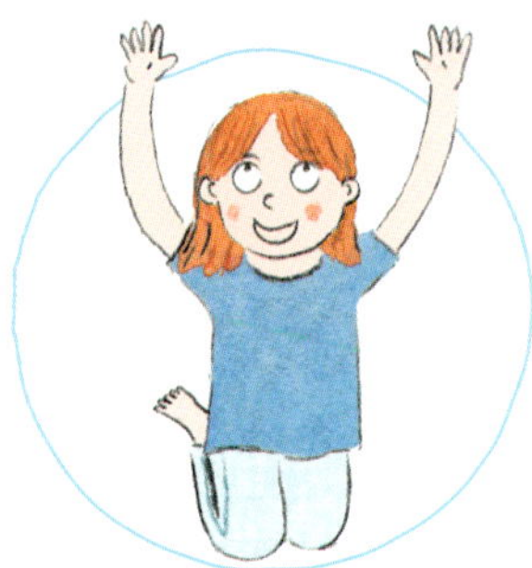

Spread your hands and lift them to the sky.

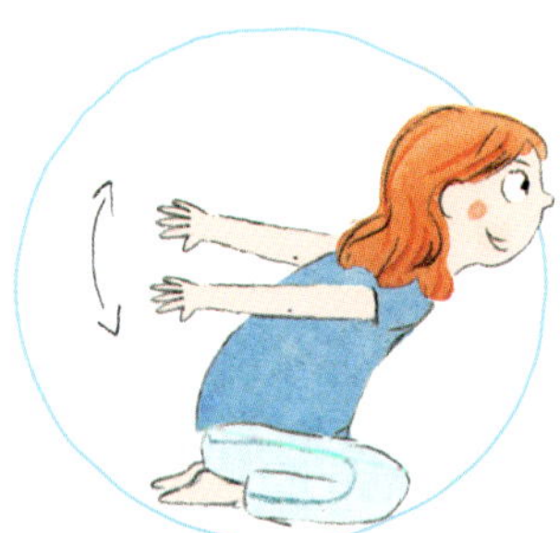

Make the upper part of your body lean in front while your hands are stretched towards the back. Spread your fingers and move your arms from the bottom to the top like the wings of a bird.

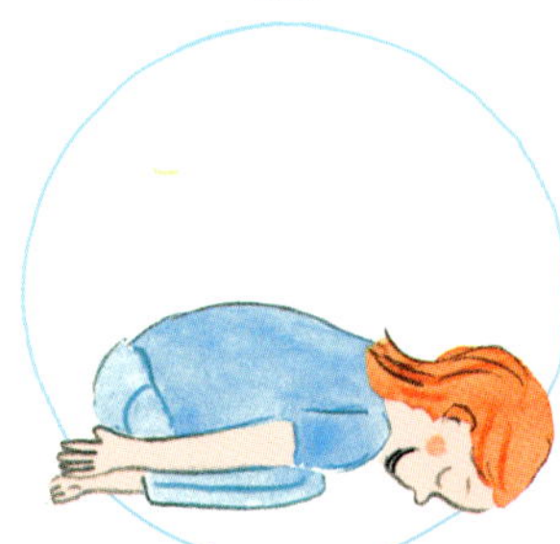

Touch your forehead to the ground, with your hands towards the back.

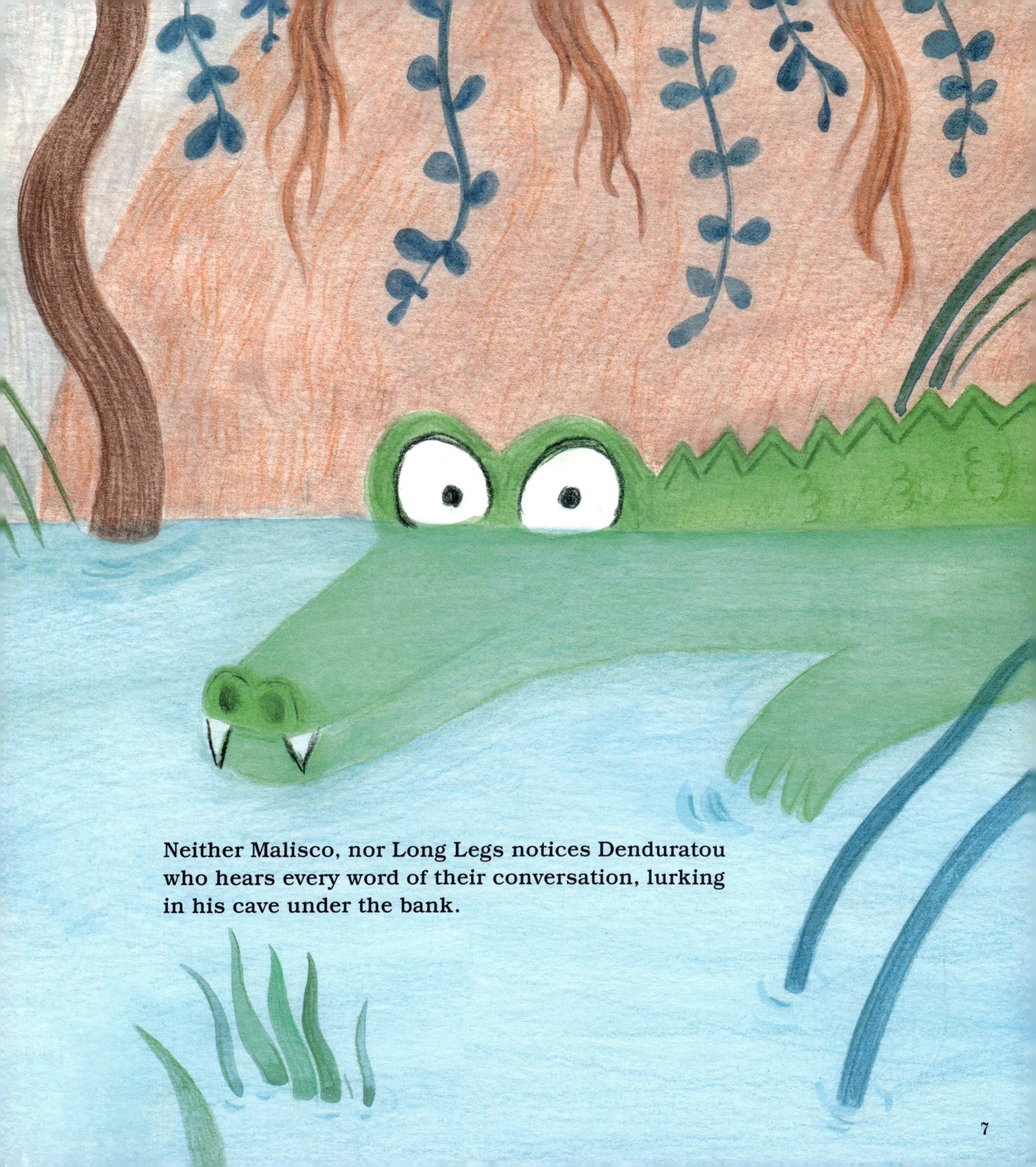

Neither Malisco, nor Long Legs notices Denduratou who hears every word of their conversation, lurking in his cave under the bank.

How lovely it is to watch wild animals from the sky!
The elephant brings his calf back to the troupe.
Hippopotami play in the muddy water.
Swift antelopes leave a cloud of golden dust behind them.
The giraffe eats the leaves from the highest branches...

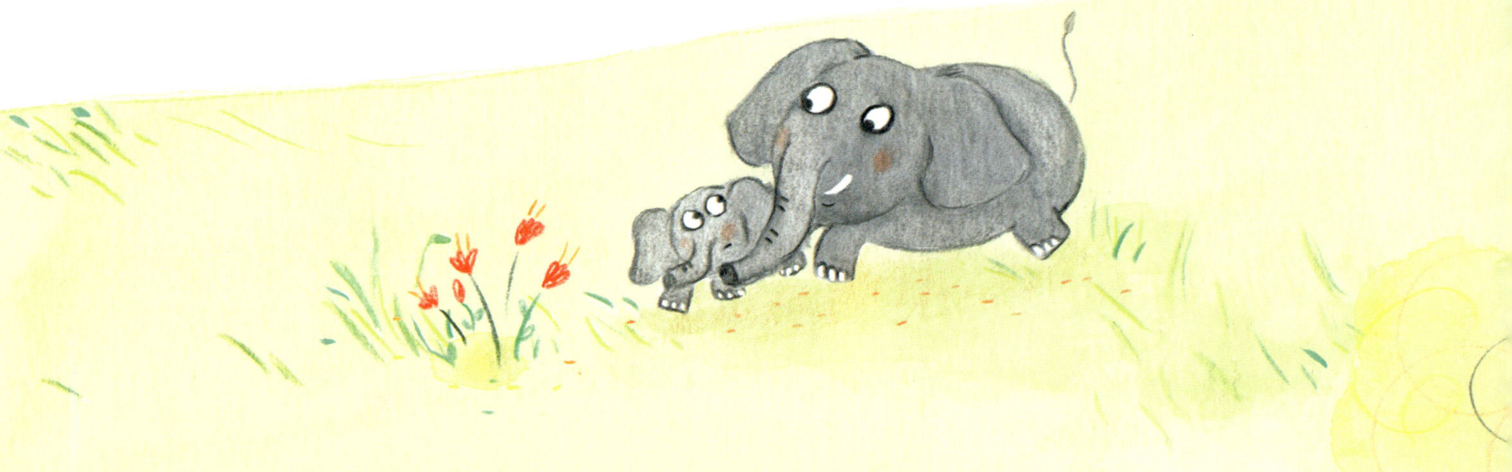

The elephant and antelope steps

Imitate the heavy step of an elephant, then walk lightly like an antelope.
Benefit: This posture develops in the child the ability to adapt while making him live through contrary physical states.

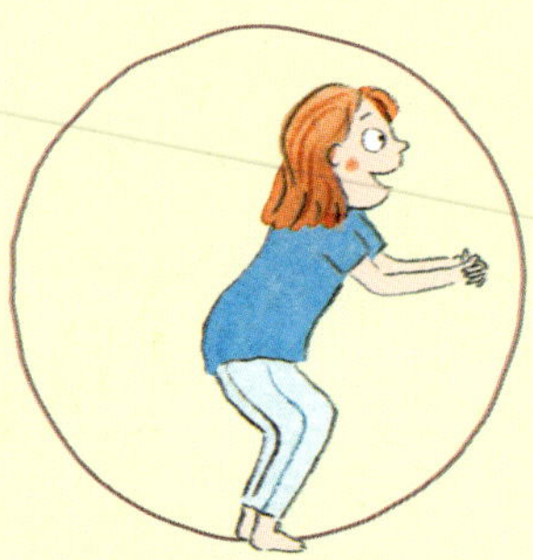

Fold the knees and dig your feet into the ground. Hold your hands in front of you and join the hands while crossing the fingers. You are now a trunk!

4 breaths

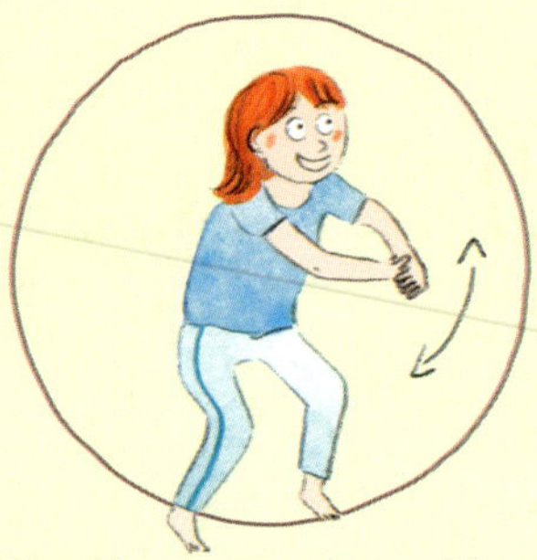

Walk with a heavy step, with your feet apart. Move your trunk in front of you while swaying your arms from the top to the bottom.

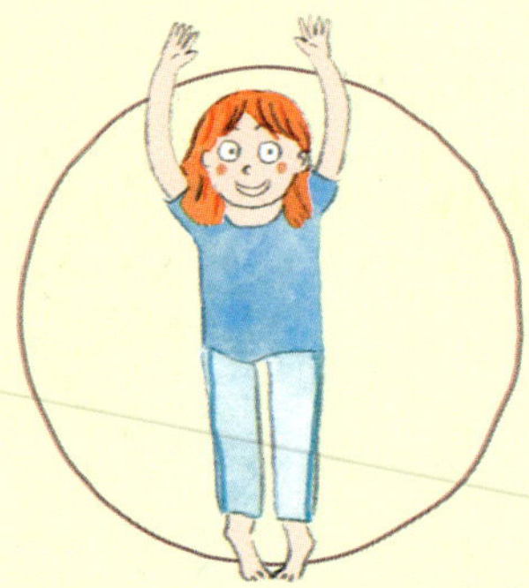

Stand straight on tiptoe and lift your hands towards the sky.

4 breaths

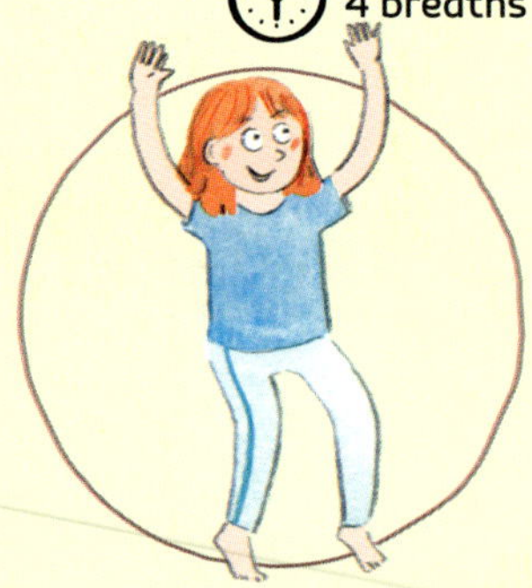

Walk on tiptoe while taking light steps.

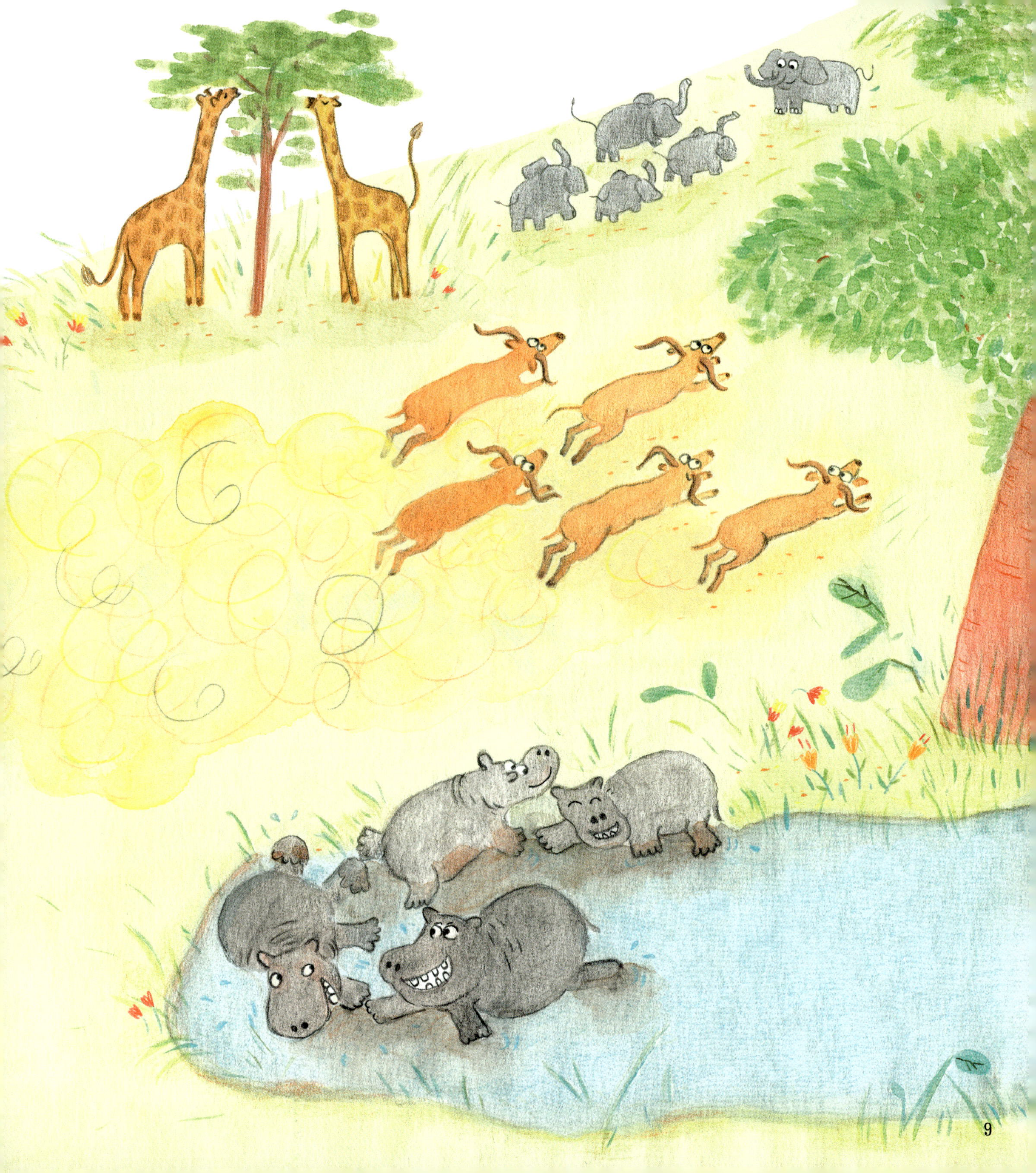

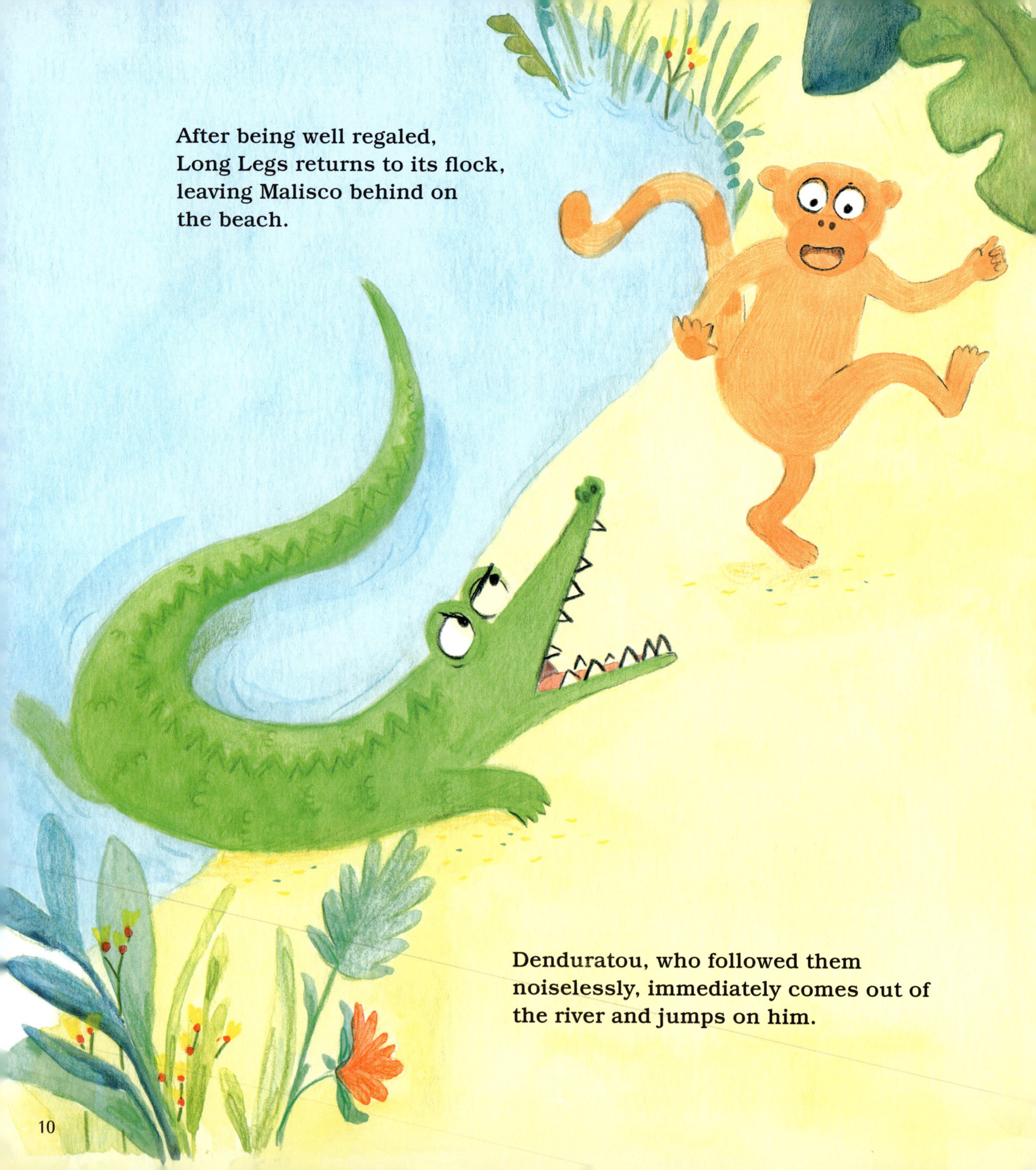

After being well regaled,
Long Legs returns to its flock,
leaving Malisco behind on
the beach.

Denduratou, who followed them
noiselessly, immediately comes out of
the river and jumps on him.

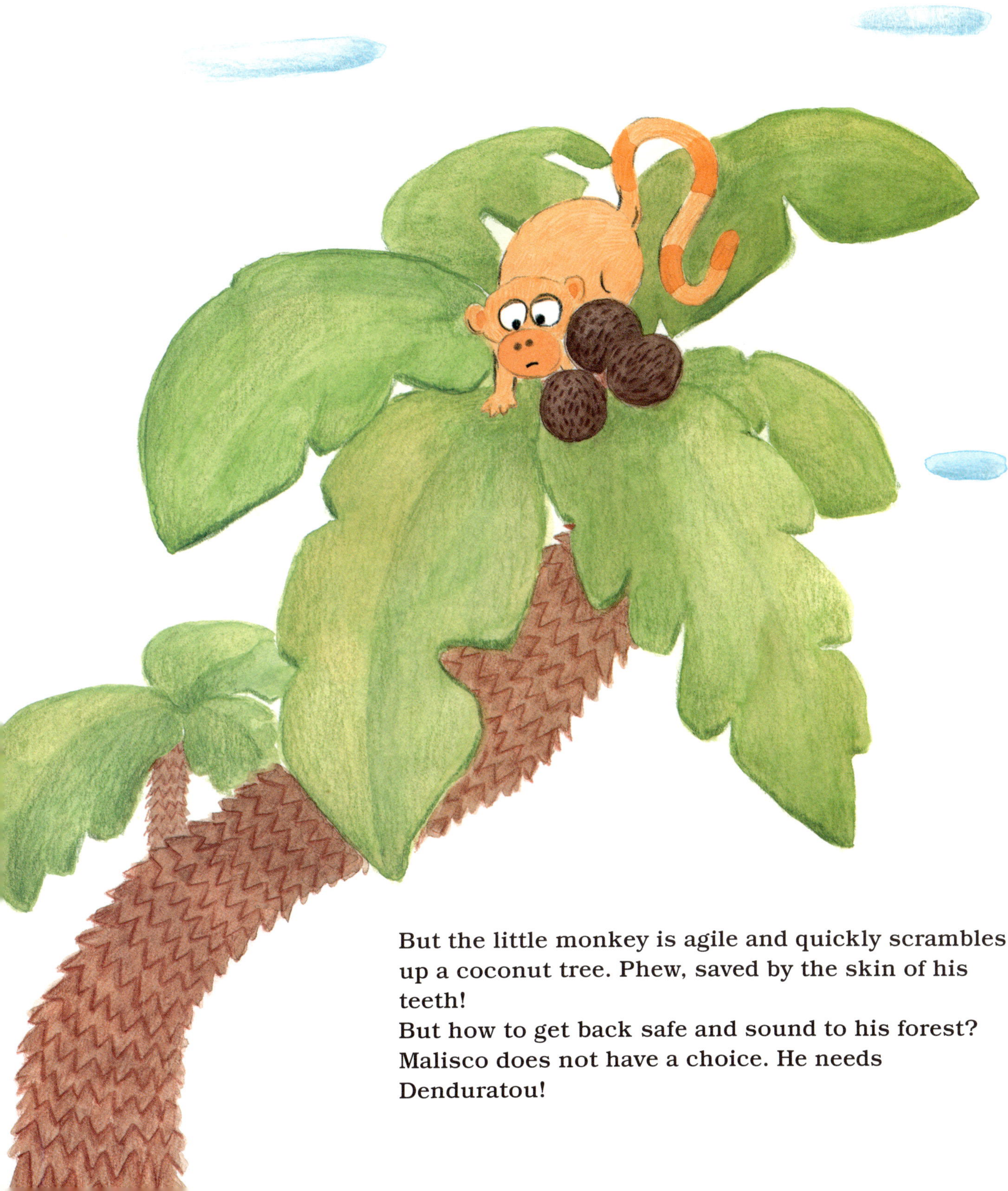

But the little monkey is agile and quickly scrambles up a coconut tree. Phew, saved by the skin of his teeth!
But how to get back safe and sound to his forest? Malisco does not have a choice. He needs Denduratou!

Fortunately, Denduratou is very stupid and Malisco is very clever. So the latter says:

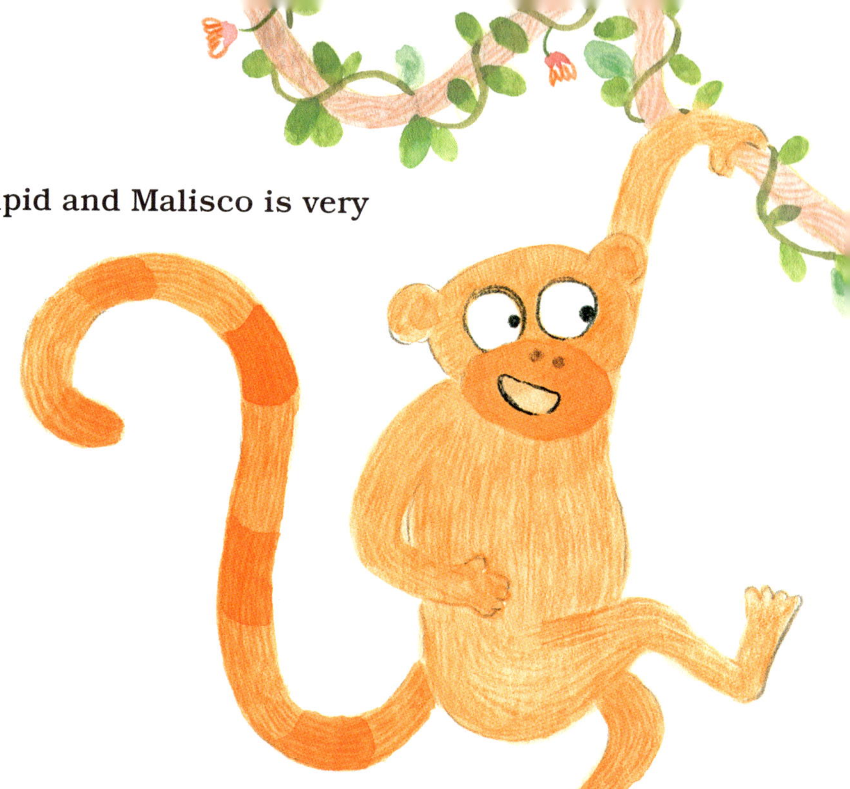

"Denduratou, I am delighted to see you! I have something to ask of you... Here you go, our Aunt Zumba has disappeared in the forest. Tomorrow, all the monkeys of the forest shall get together to plead with the Spirit of the forest to return her to us. But you know the Grand Spirit: without crying or tears, no wish shall be granted!

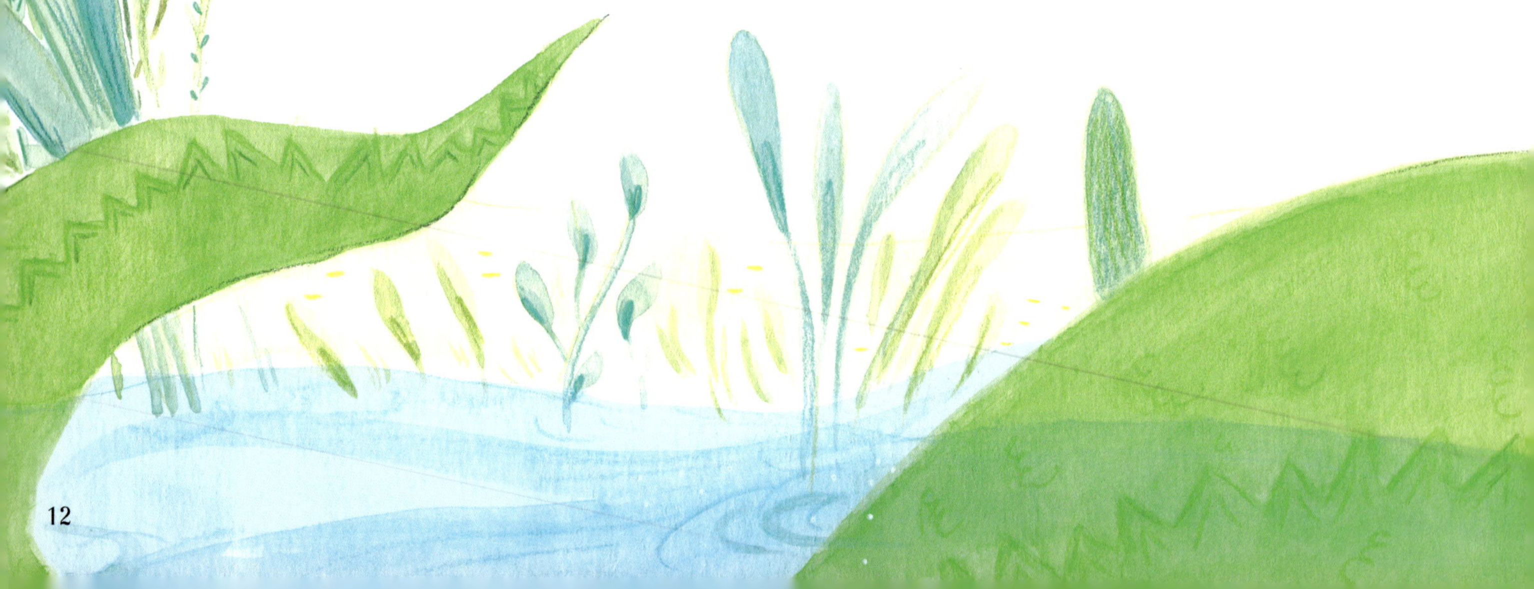

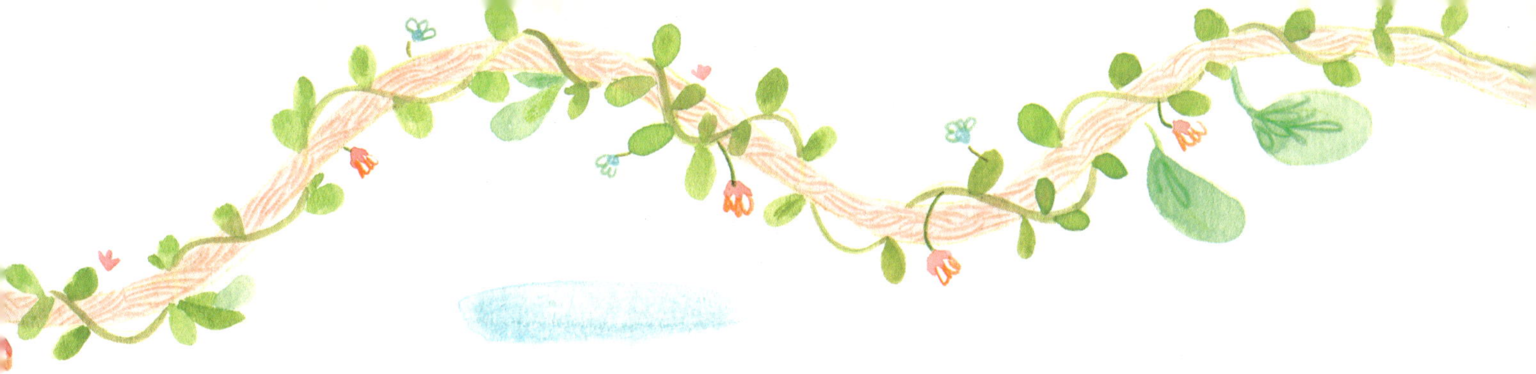

"But we monkeys shall not be able to cry. No chance! You see, old Aunt Zumba always gave us rotten bananas to eat when we visited her.

"So you understand, we are not grieving. But you crocodiles, you are able to cry when you want. Isn't that so?"

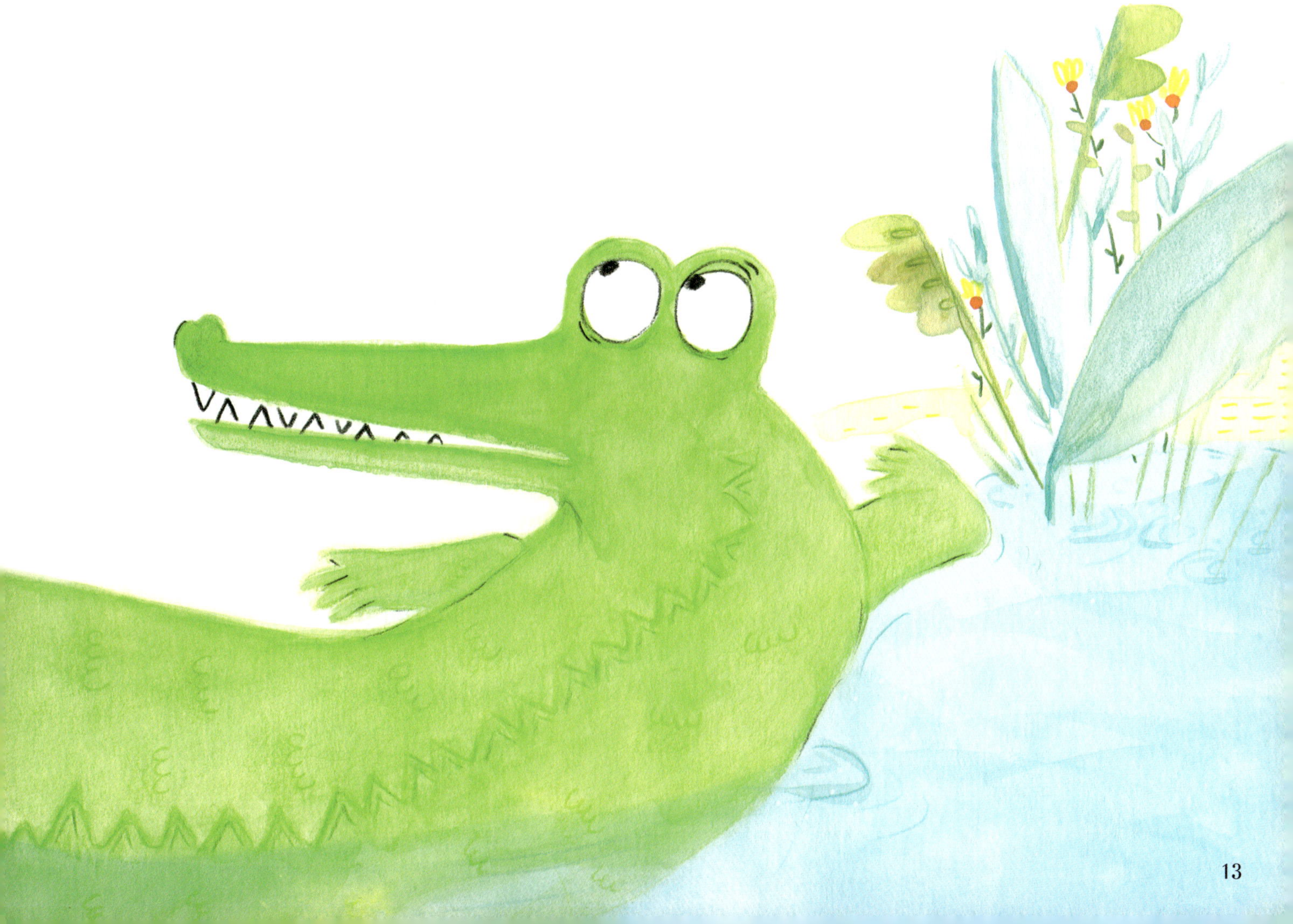

Taken aback at this talk, the crocodile answers without thinking:
"You are right! That's even our speciality. Look..."
He blinks his eyelids and immediately tears stream down his cheeks in torrents. This is what one calls crocodile tears.

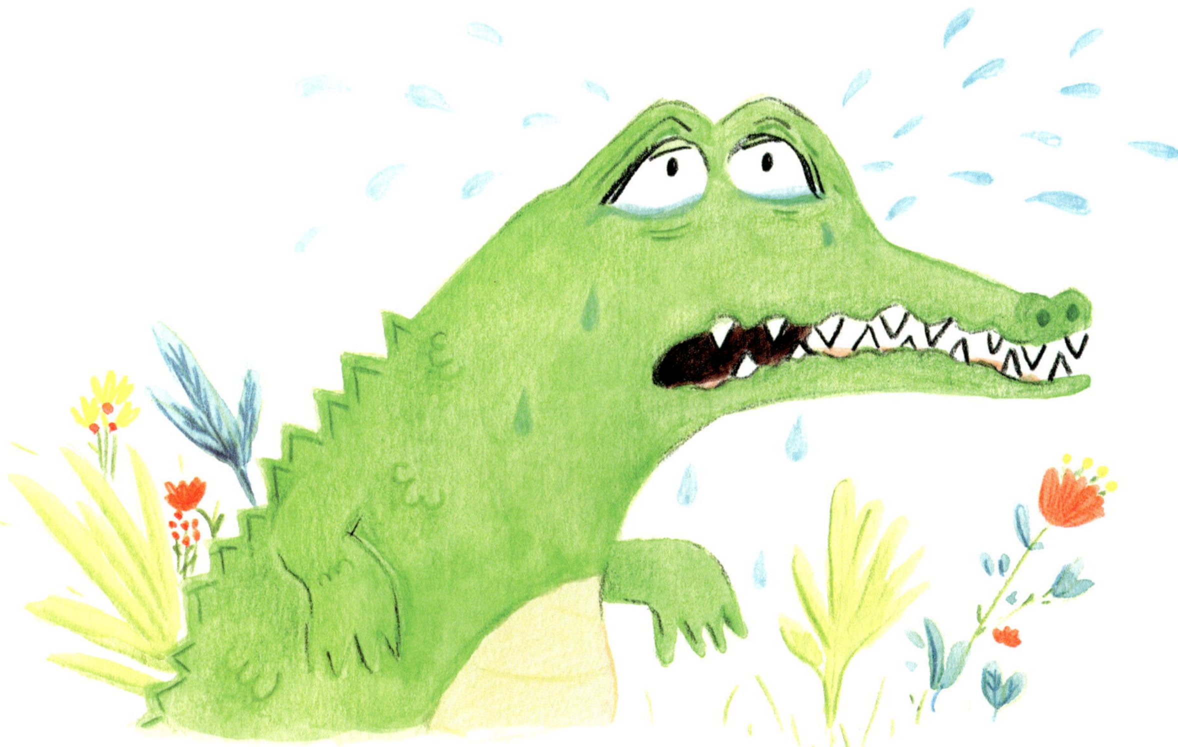

Denduratou's tears

You too shed crocodile tears!

Benefits: This exercise tones up breathing and softens the diaphragm while providing energy.

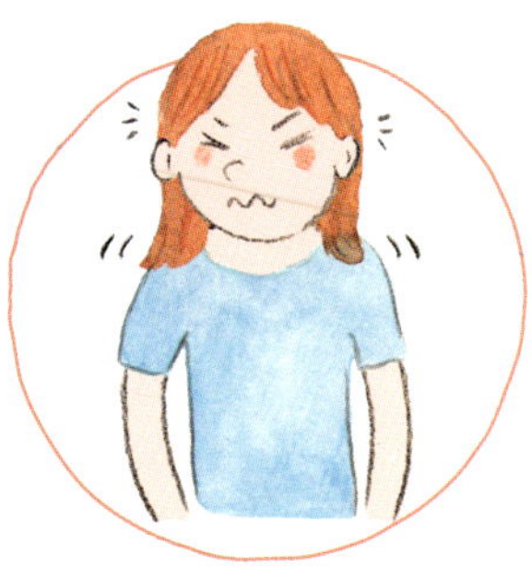

Take many short breaths while inflating the chest: pretend to cry like a crocodile!

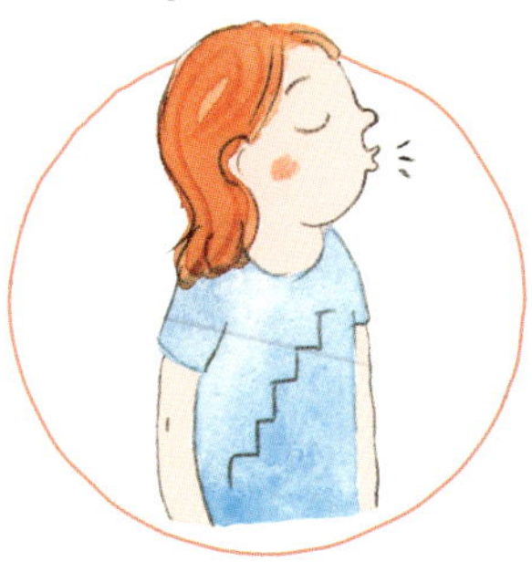

Imagine your breath is climbing stairs: feel how it climbs higher, and higher...

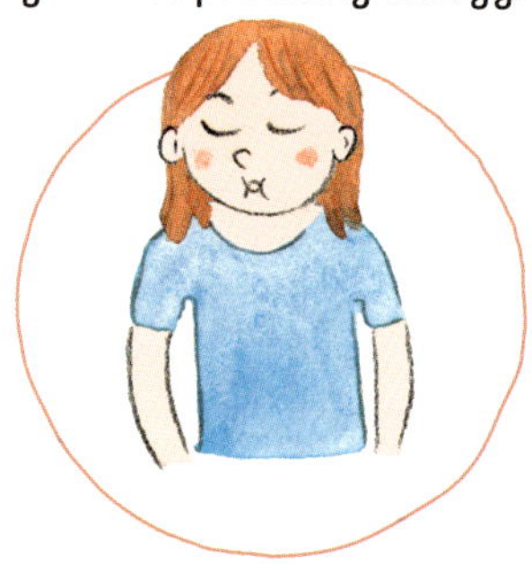

Let out a deep sigh. Repeat all the steps two times.

Malisco bursts with joy:
"Marvellous! This is exactly what we need: false grief and real tears. Could you give some to each of us? We could offer these to the Grand Spirit."

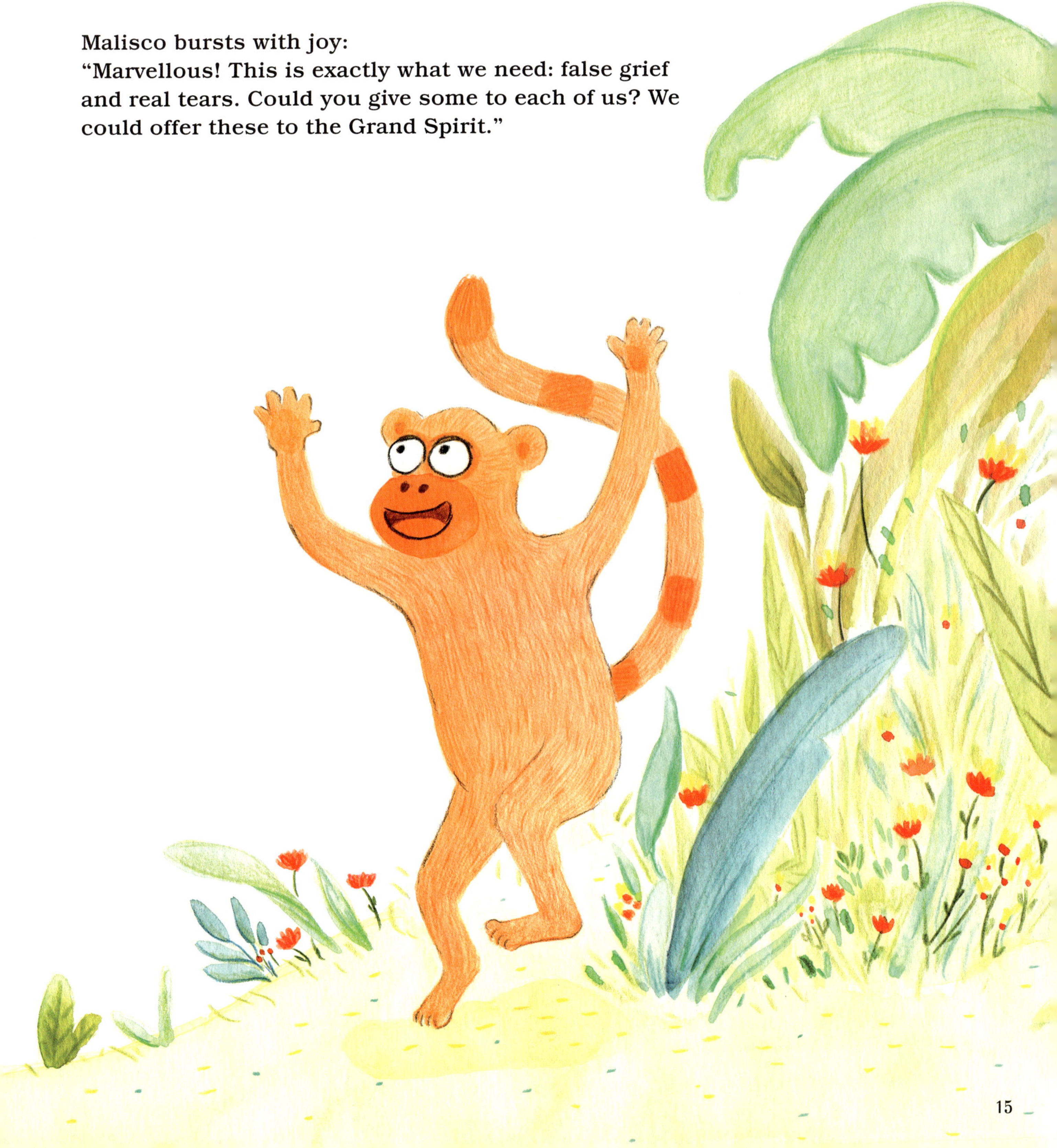

In the pea-sized brain inside his fat head of a crocodile, Denduratou suddenly realises that instead of one monkey, he can polish off an entire tribe.

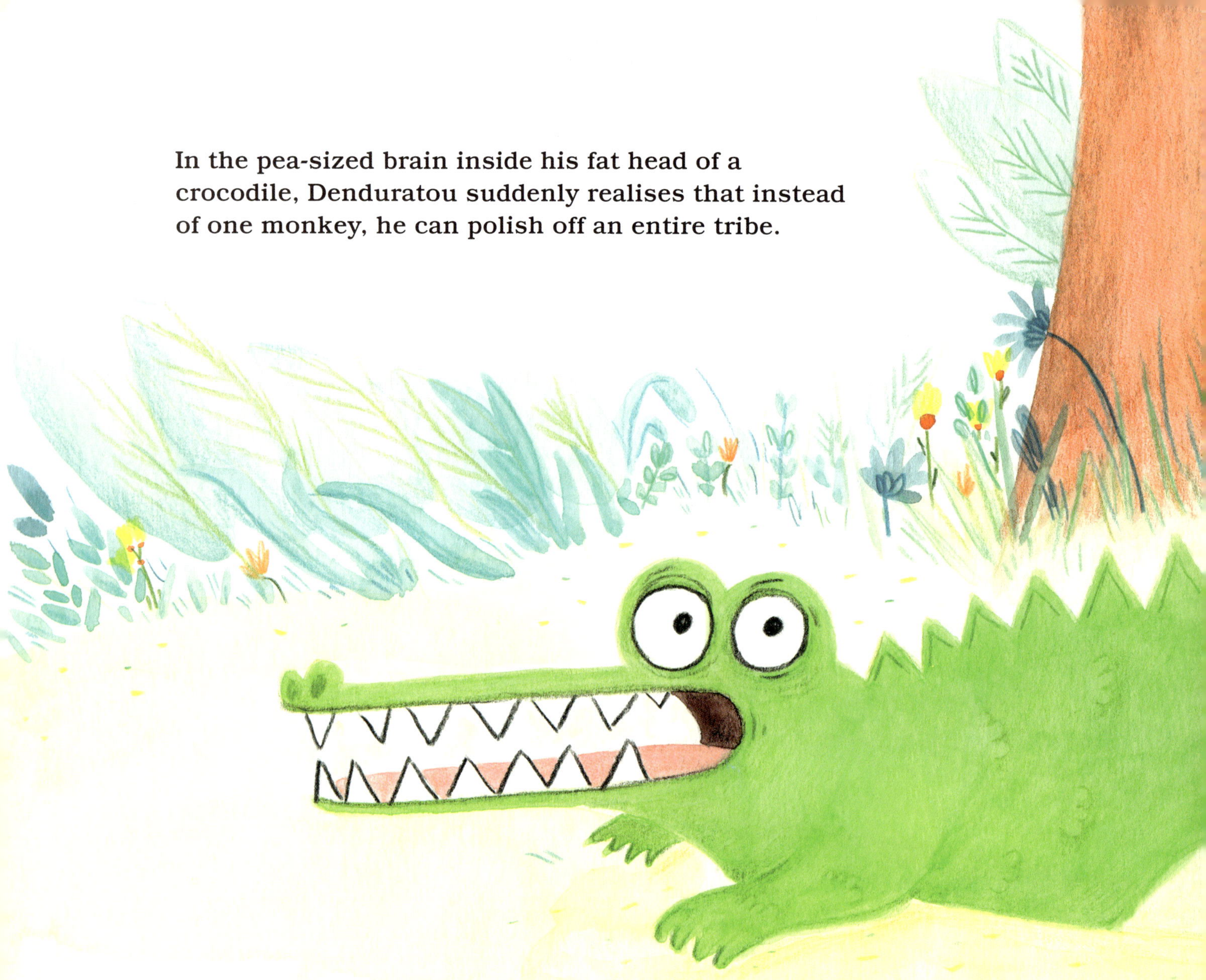

So he too hatches a plan:
"In that case, it's best that you all come along one after another since I too need to replenish my bag of tears. And when each monkey gets his share of tears, he can wait in the cave with the others. And all of you can leave together after that."

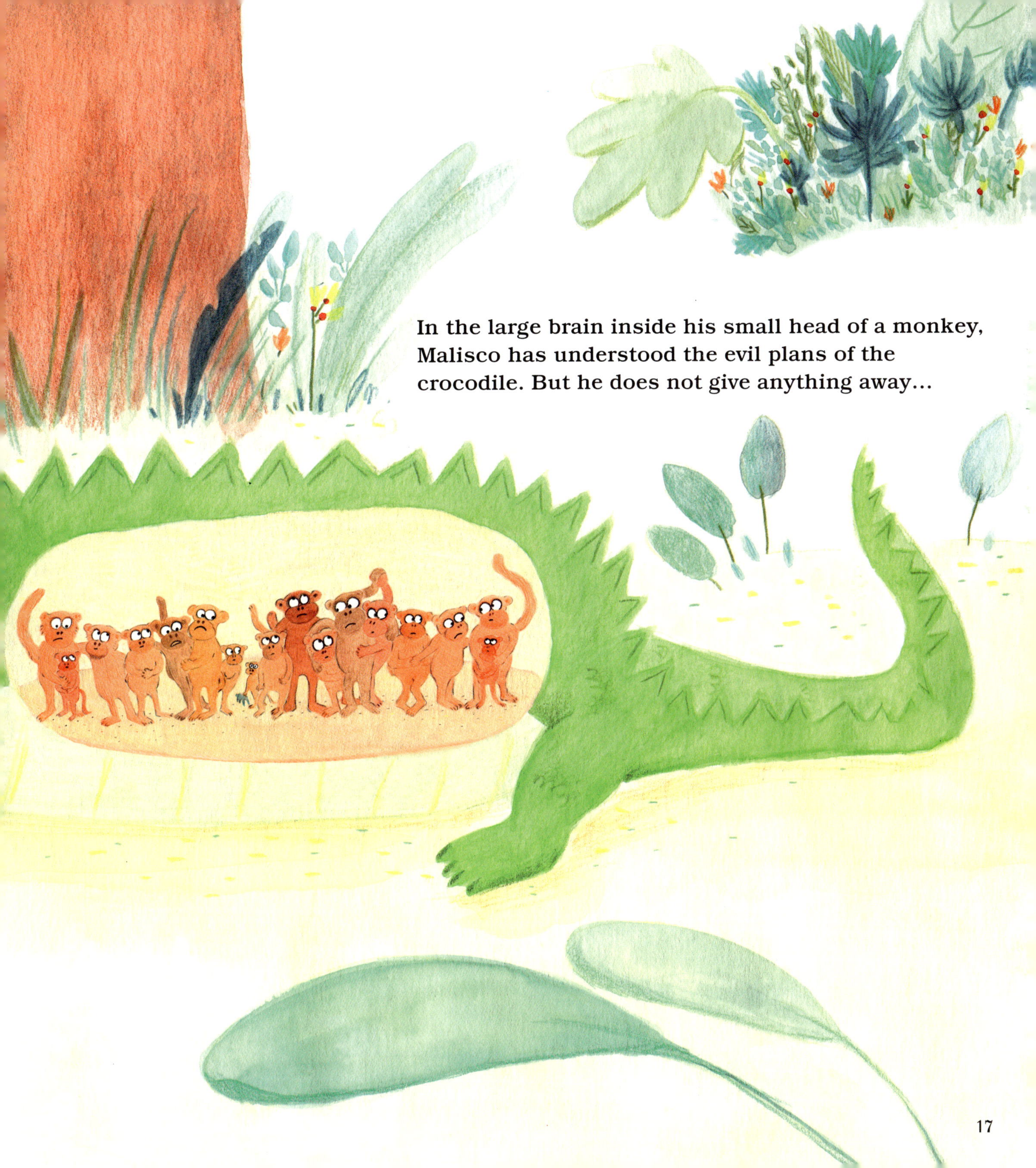

In the large brain inside his small head of a monkey, Malisco has understood the evil plans of the crocodile. But he does not give anything away...

“That is very nice of you! While we are at it, could you help me transport coconuts to the island for the grand feast in honour of the Grand Spirit? You could leave them on the bank and my brothers could carry them to the forest.”

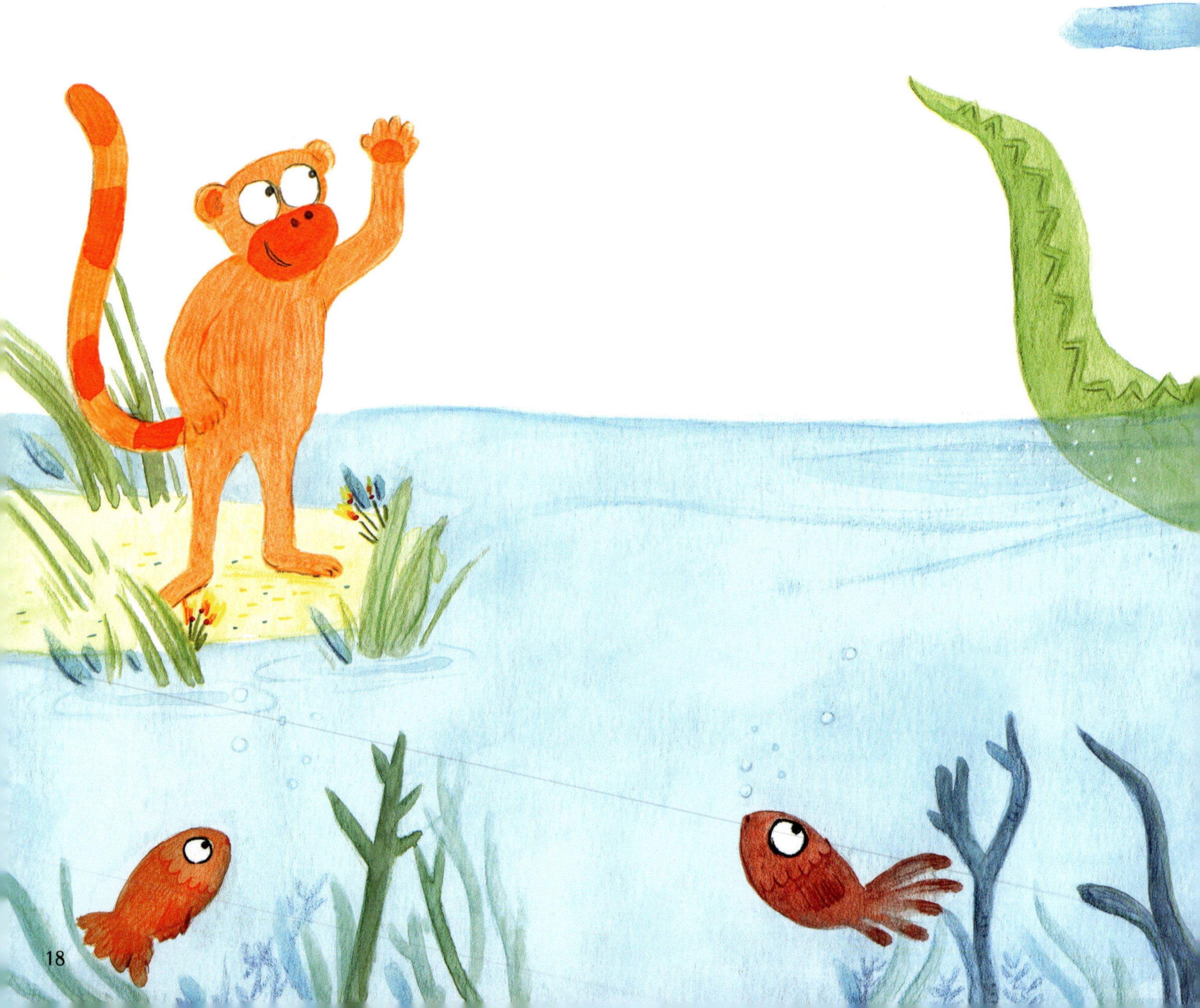

Not thinking beyond the sumptuous meal that awaits him, Denduratou replies:
"Stuff my mouth with as many coconuts as it can carry. I shall make as many trips as you wish."

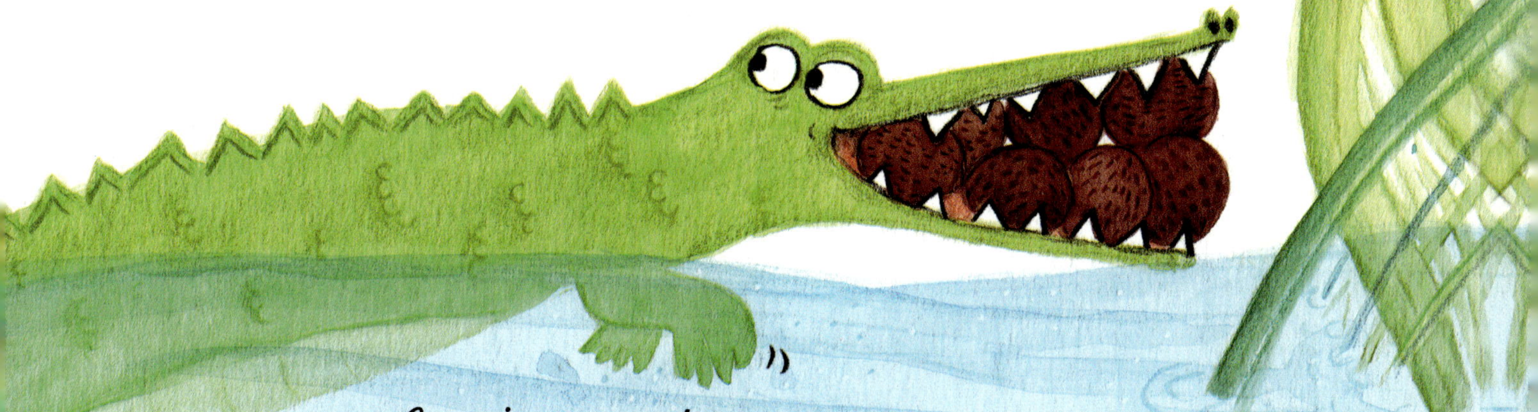

Carrying coconuts

What if you were to help Denduratou carry the coconuts?
Benefits: This posture improves the head's position in maintaining balance while walking and strengthens the thighs.

4 breaths

3 breaths

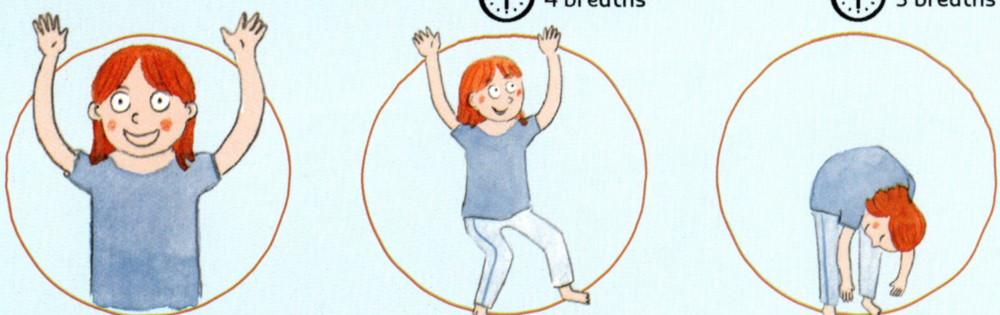

While standing, lift your hands and spread your fingers: you are carrying a huge coconut.

Fold your legs and walk. Look ahead and keep your back straight so as not to drop the coconut.

Lean in front, with your legs stretched. Let the upper part of your body drop towards the ground.

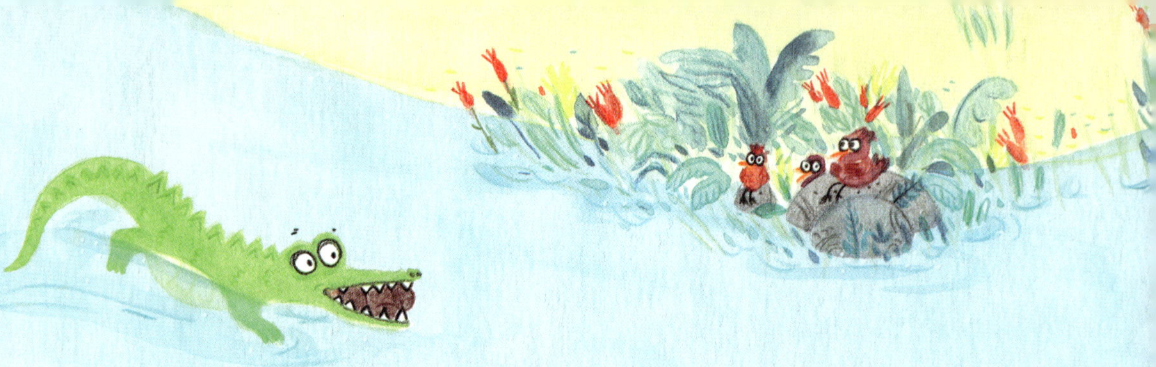

Well! He goes back and forth...

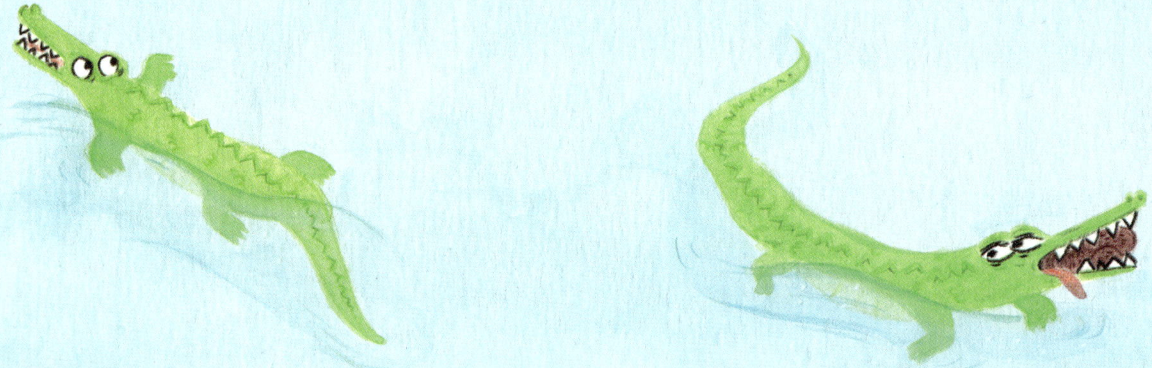

During this time, taking advantage of the situation, Malisco eats all that he loves on the island. It's party time!

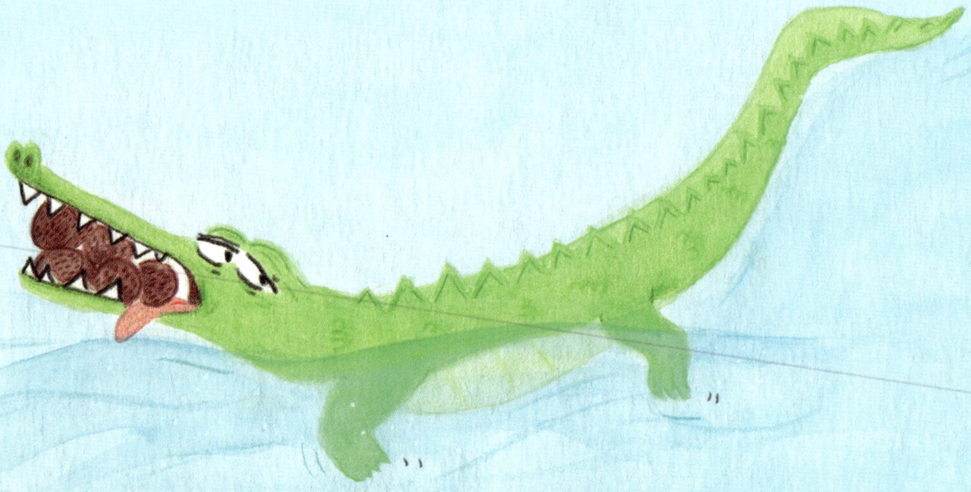

Thereafter, he plays in the trees, swaying from one branch to another with Centano, the snake. Oh, how happy he is!

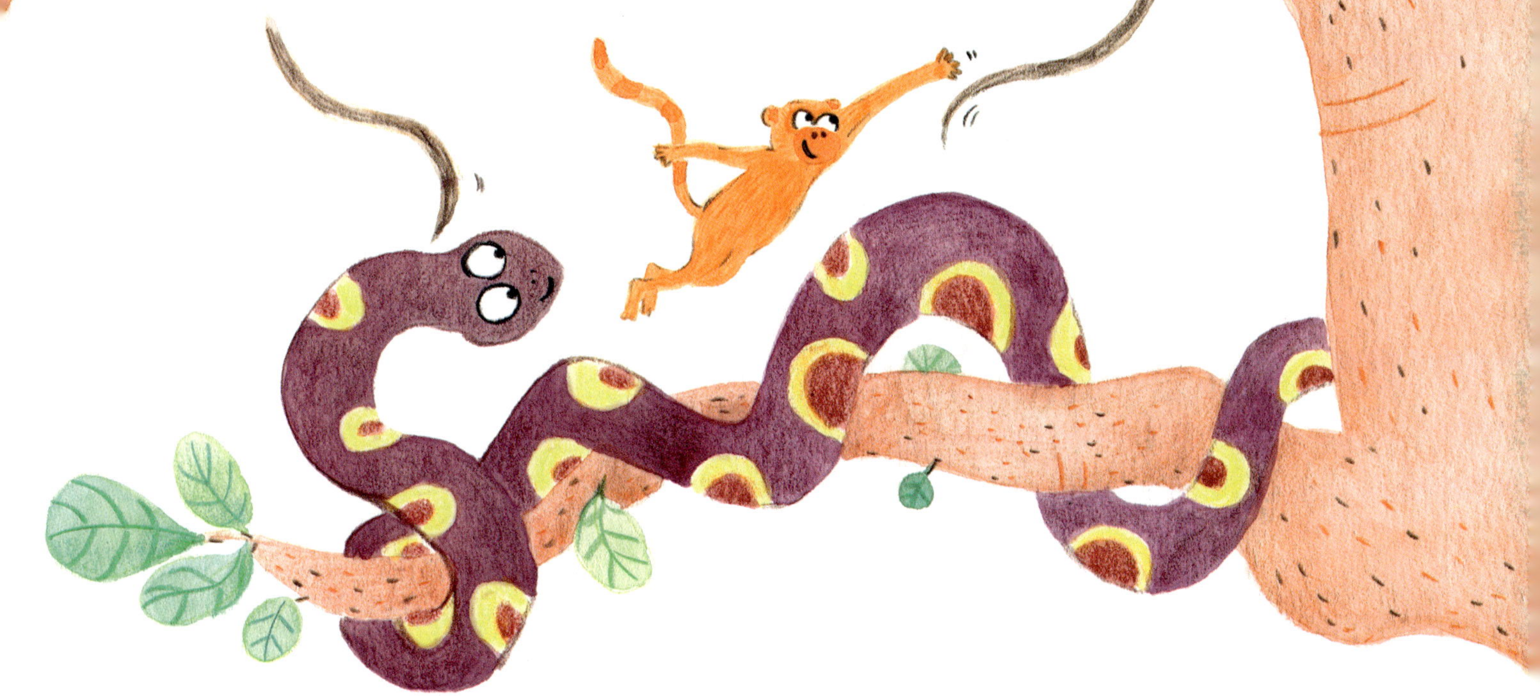

The snake

Now have fun being a snake.

Benefits : This posture teaches the child to straighten himself with the help of the ground while strengthening the hands and the lower body.

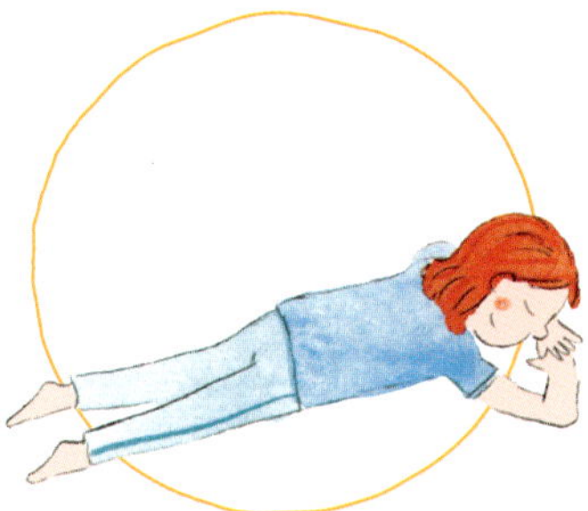

Lie down on the ground and place your forehead on your hands that are on top of each other.

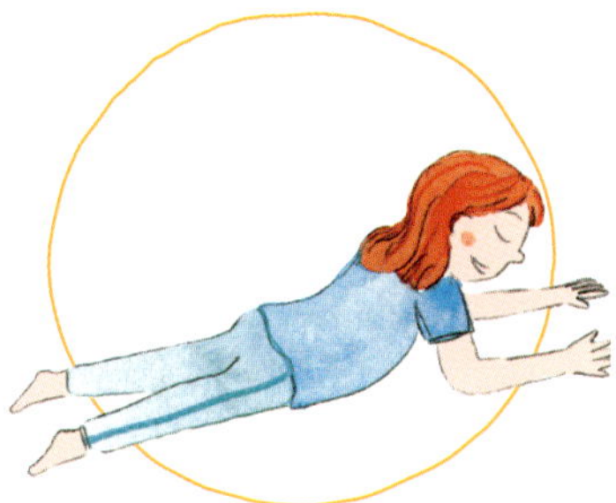

Lift yourself up with the help of your elbows and straighten your bust while you keep your stomach on the ground.

3 breaths

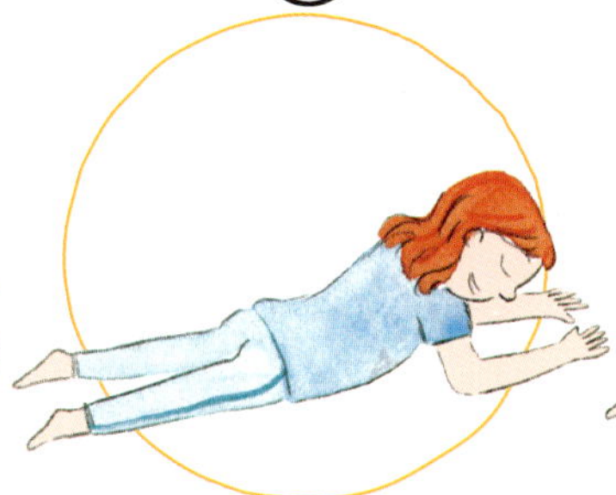

Bring your chin towards your throat.

4 breaths

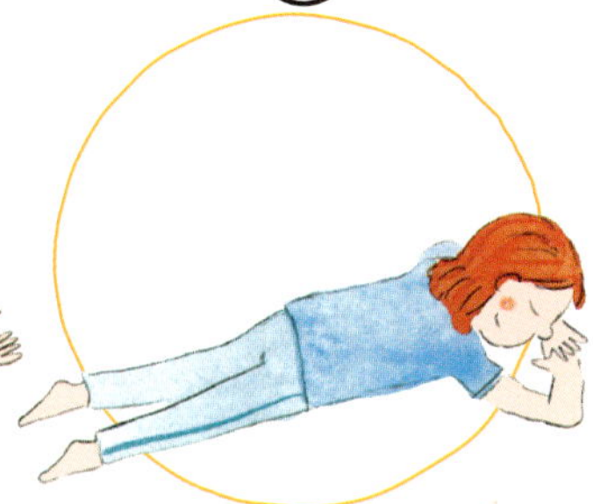

Get back to the original position.

On the last round, the crocodile takes Malisco on his back. As the latter balances himself, he looks like the sail of a boat.

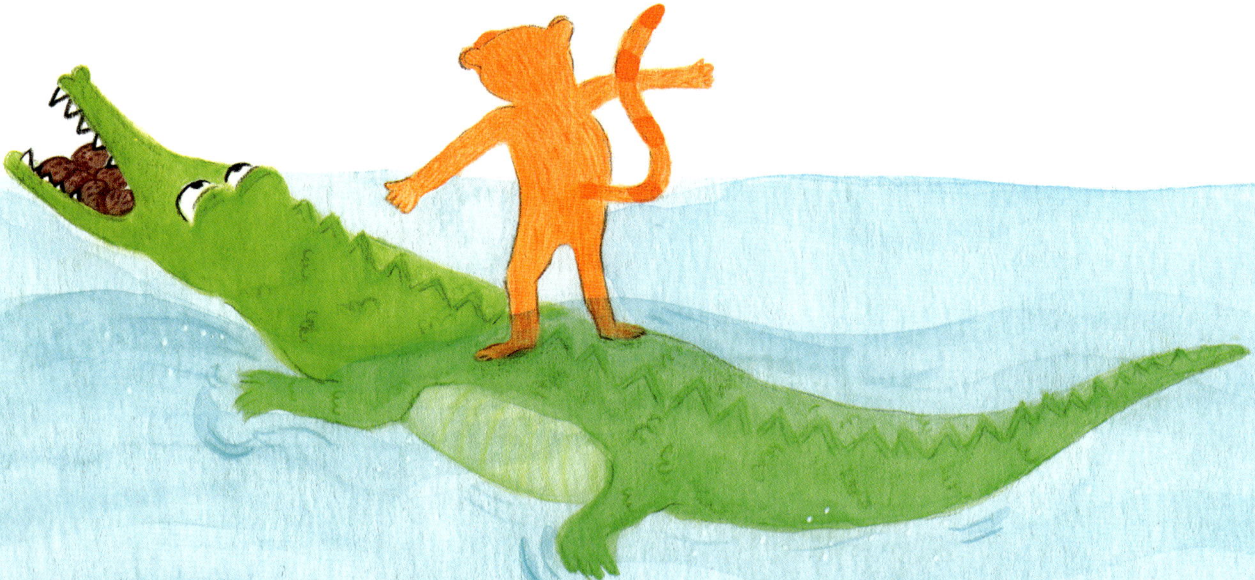

The sail

Like the sail, the wind pushes you in the back.

Benefit: This posture teaches the child to play with the elements while associating the wind with the lightness of the body.

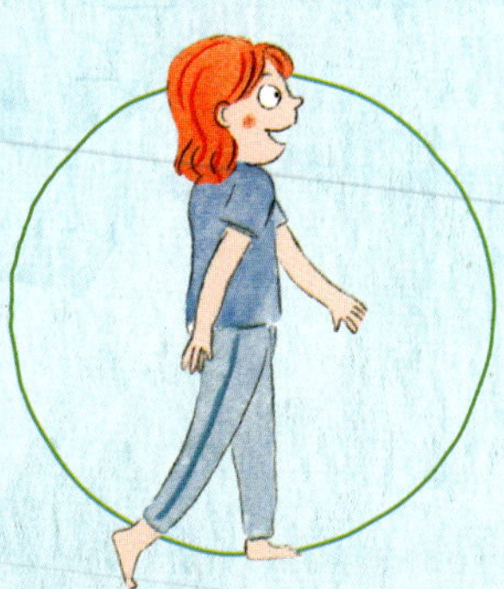

While standing, glide one leg towards the back with the tip of the foot. Support yourself on the foot in front.

3 breaths

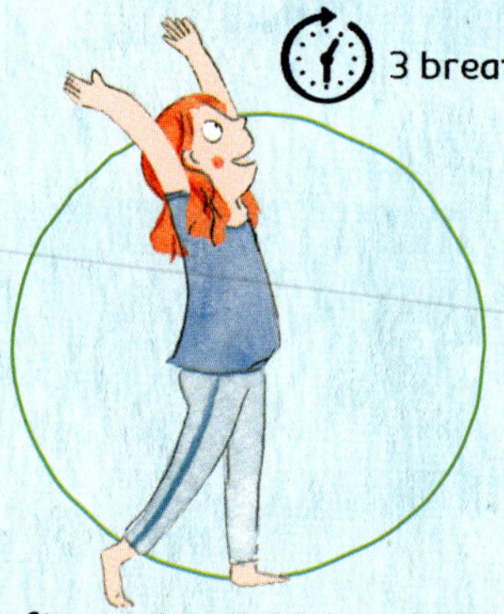

Lift your hands high and a bit towards the back. Thrust out your pelvis and stretch your back to form a nice curve.

4 breaths

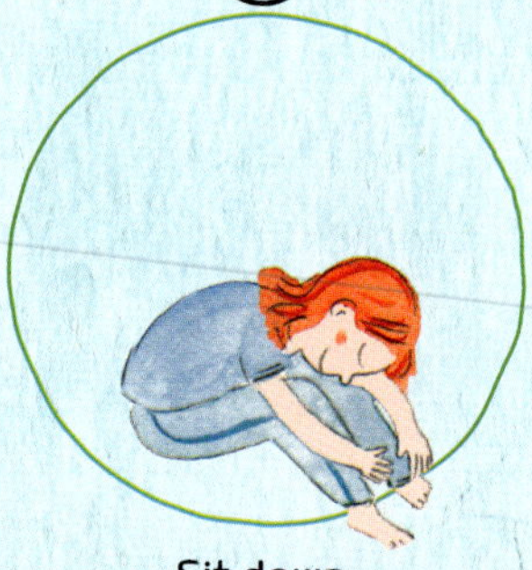

Sit down, fold your legs and place your head on your folded knees.

What a funny boat!
The fish gape at it.

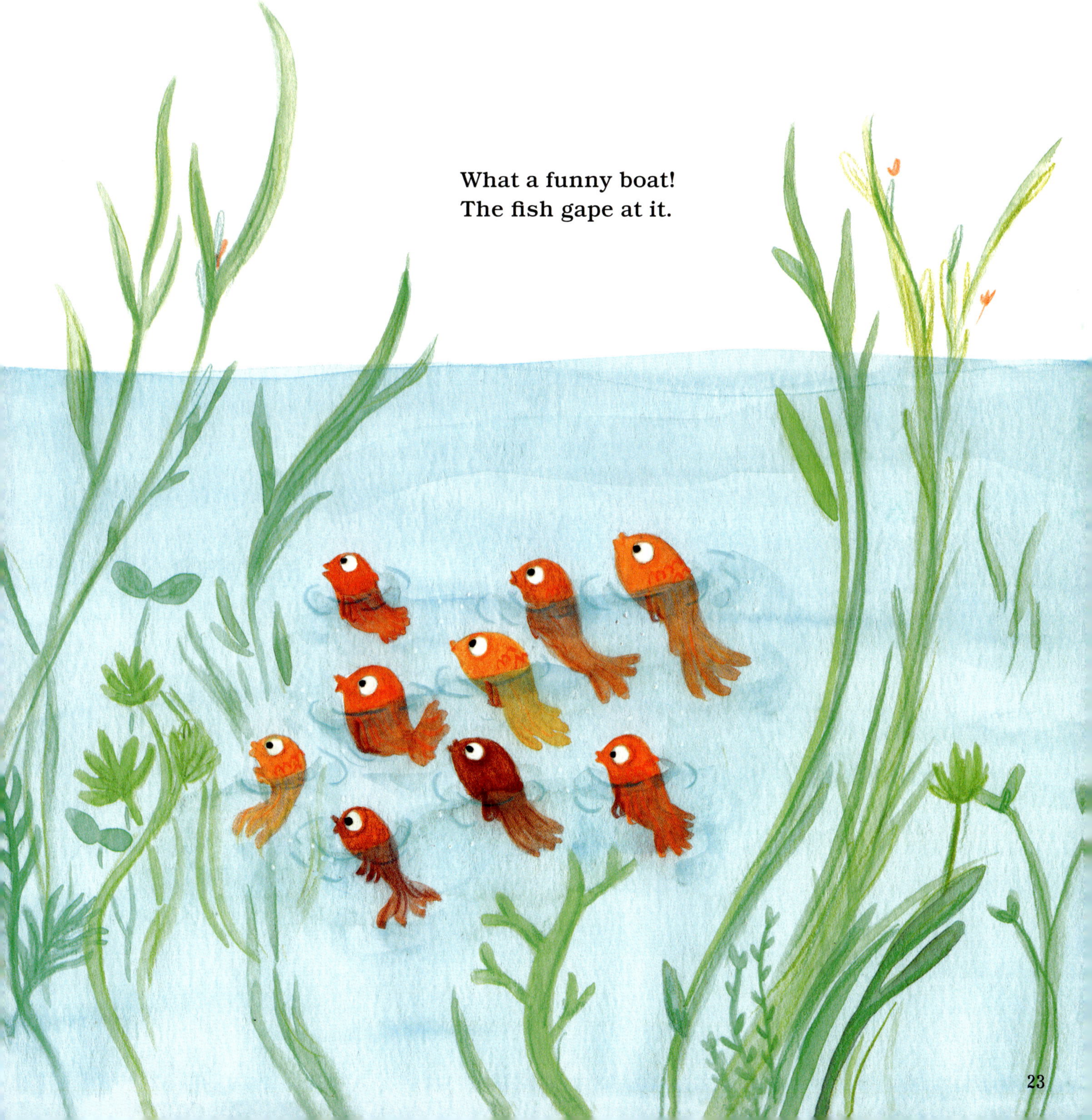

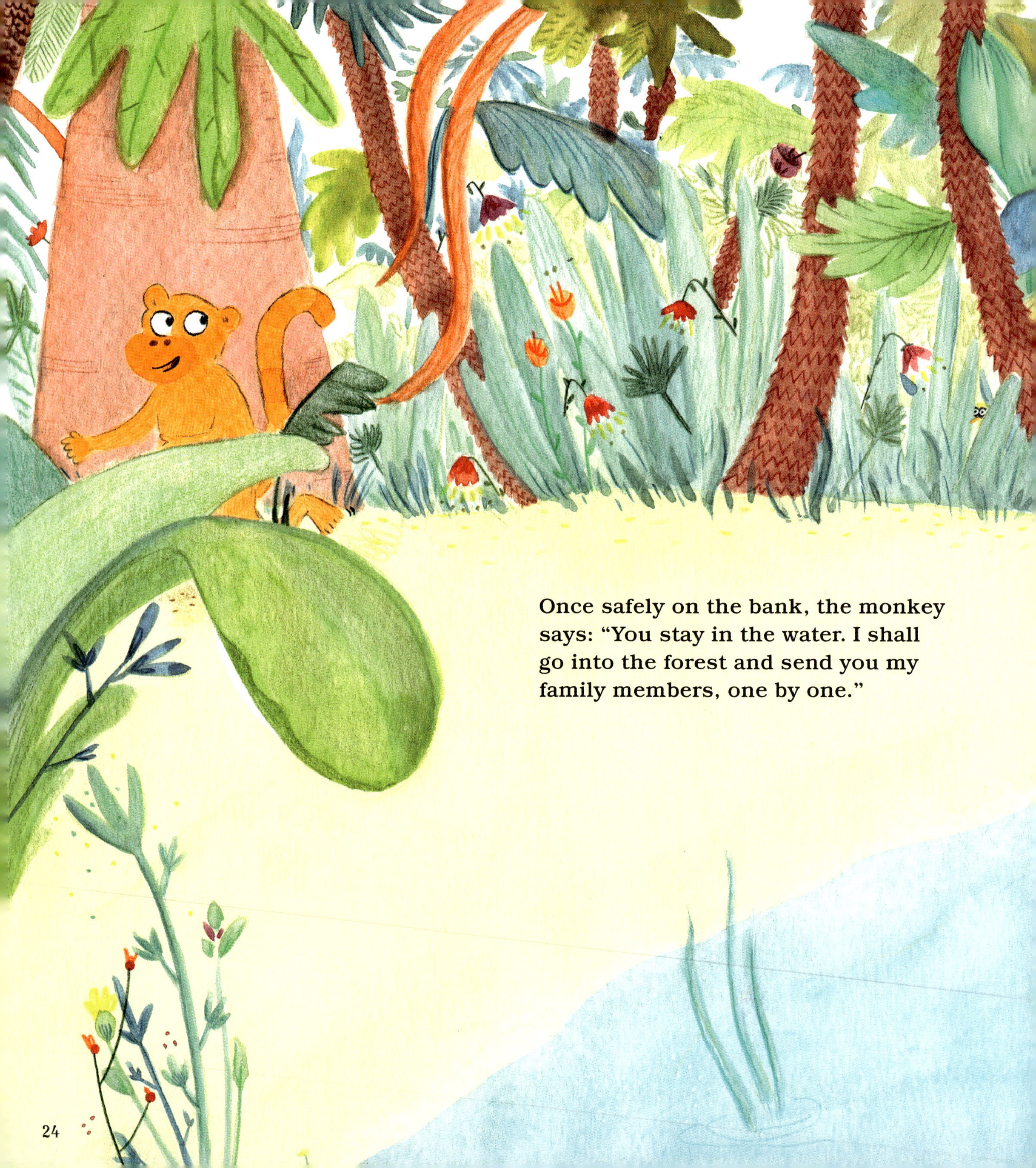

Once safely on the bank, the monkey says: “You stay in the water. I shall go into the forest and send you my family members, one by one.”

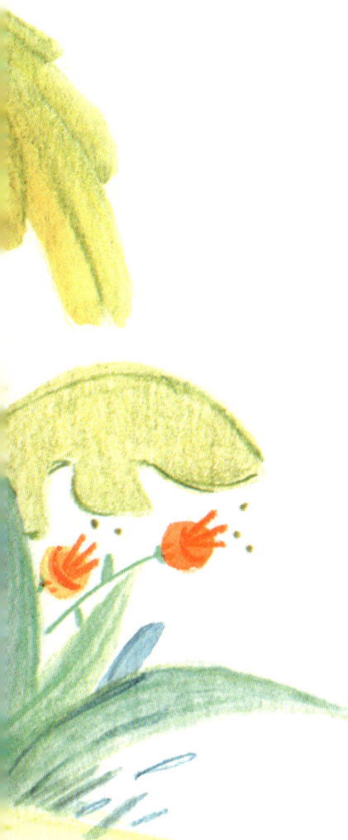

An impatient Denduratou trembles.
He waits, and waits, and waits...

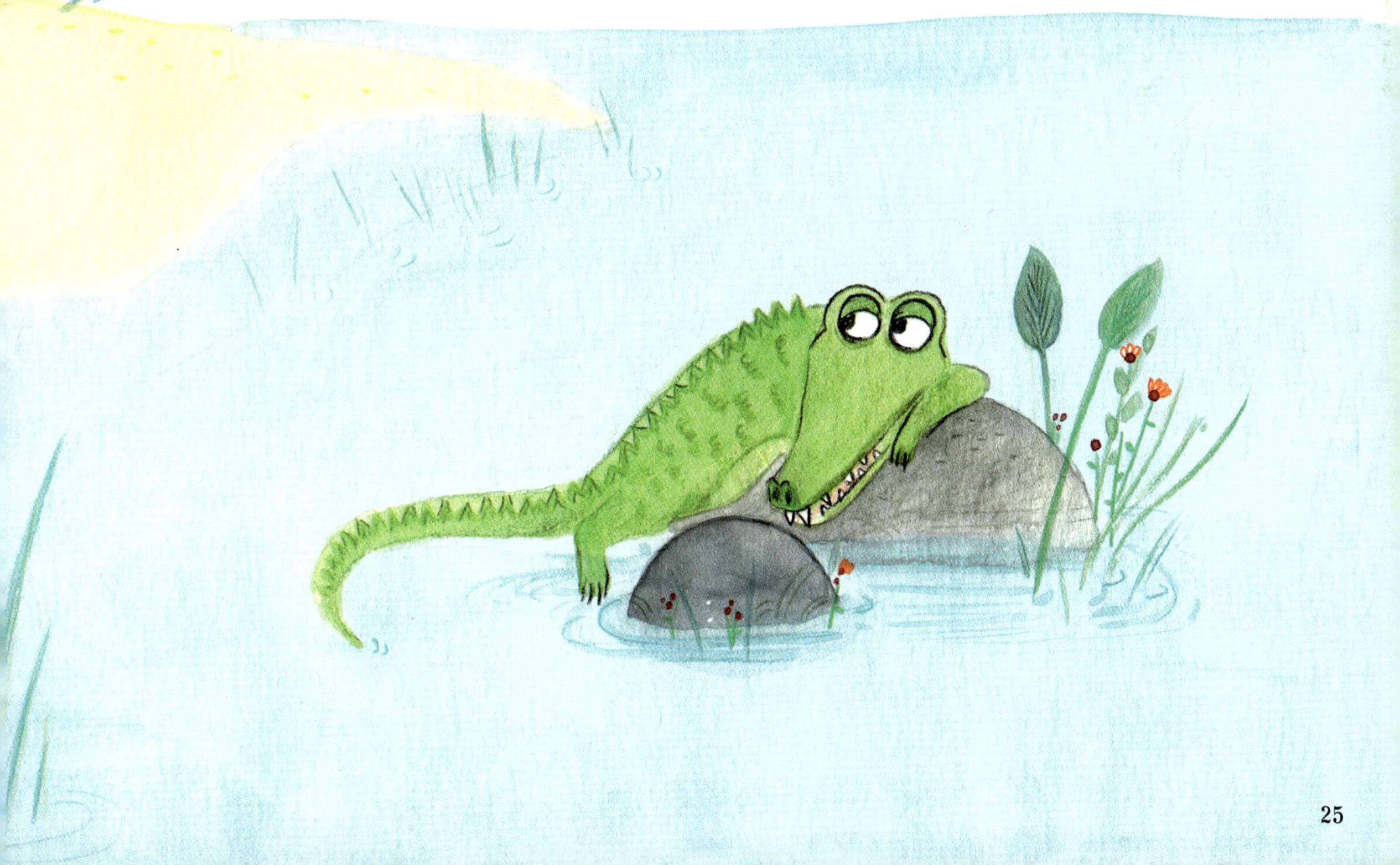

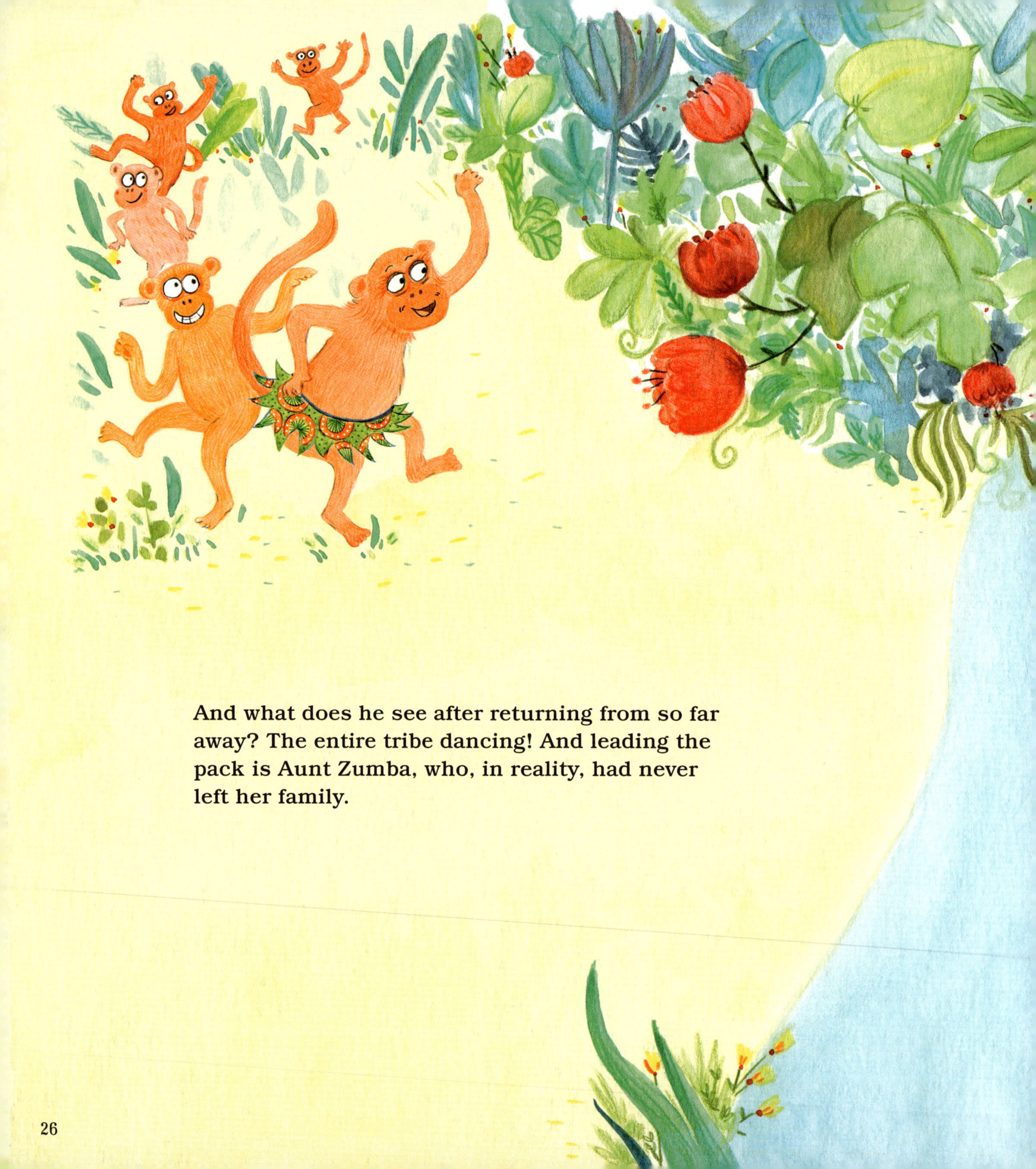

And what does he see after returning from so far away? The entire tribe dancing! And leading the pack is Aunt Zumba, who, in reality, had never left her family.

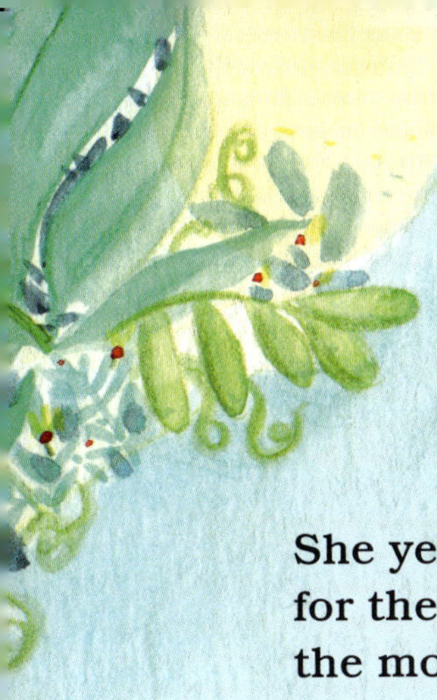

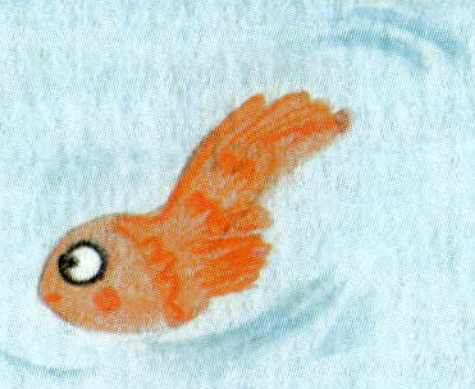

She yells at him from a distance, however: “Thanks for the coconuts, Denduratou! Without doubt, you are the most helpful crocodile in entire Africa. You have made us crrrrrrry while laughing.”

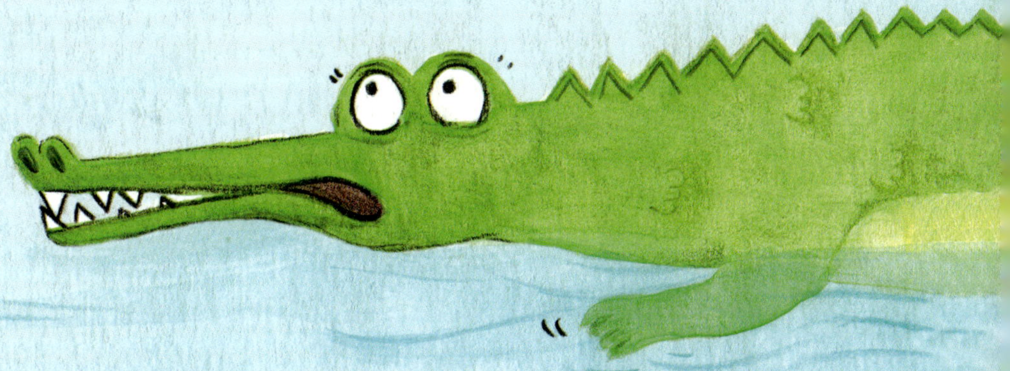

Crying while laughing

Malisco’s story has made you laugh, hasn’t it? Prove it.

Benefit: While unwinding the diaphragm, this respiratory exercise helps de-stress while provoking laughter.

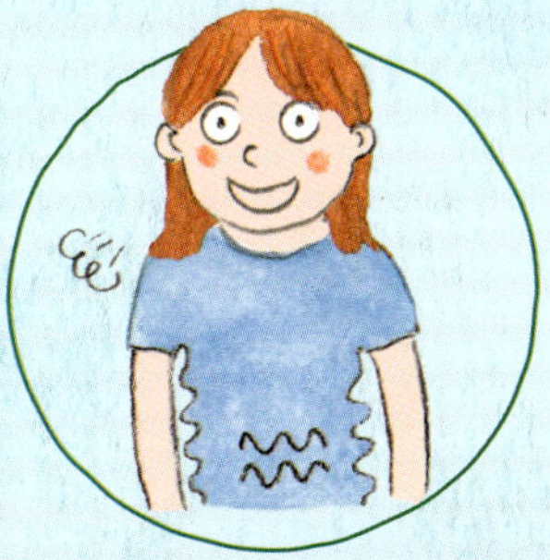

Exhale a few times while shaking your stomach as though you are dying to laugh. The air coming out of your nose makes a noise.

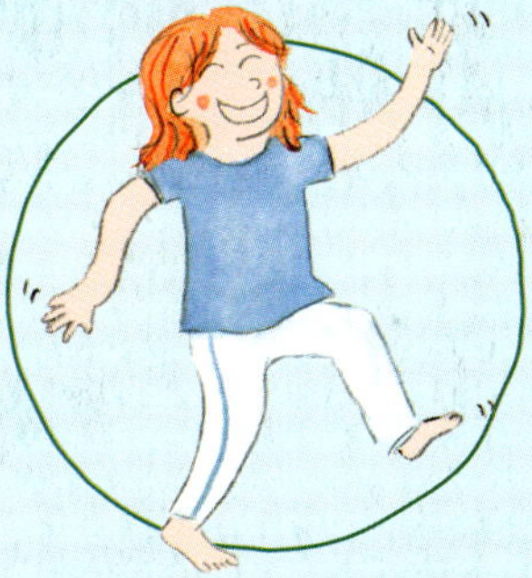

Now laugh and dance!

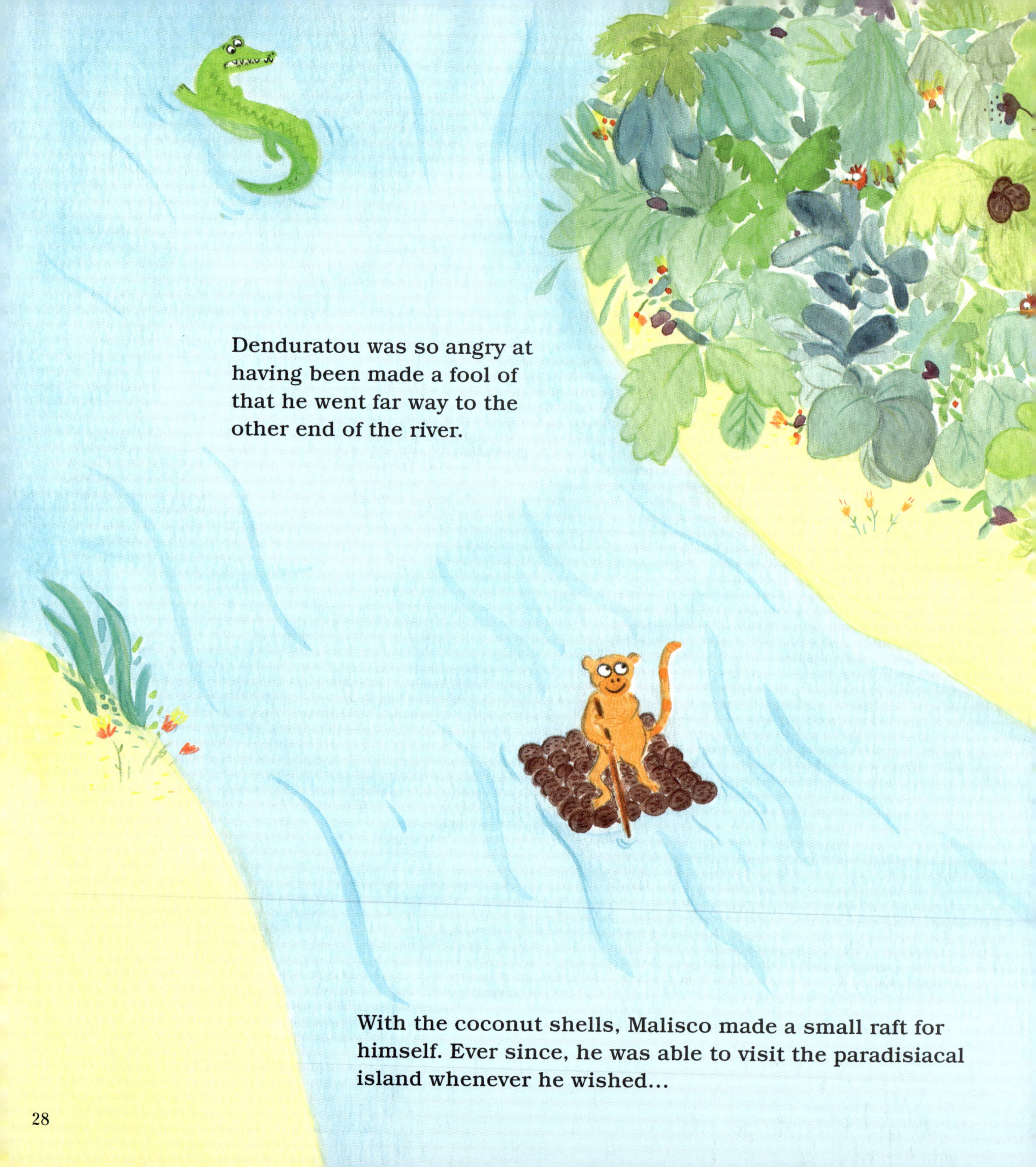

Denduratou was so angry at having been made a fool of that he went far way to the other end of the river.

With the coconut shells, Malisco made a small raft for himself. Ever since, he was able to visit the paradisiacal island whenever he wished...

Relaxation

The story is finished. Now you shall relax.

- **Choose a quiet place, with cushions and stuffed toys (or a blanket for instance).**
- **Dim the lights.**
- **Make yourself comfortable and read these texts out to the child.**
- **Speak slowly and softly.**

If the child is a bit reluctant and finds it difficult to calm down, do not insist on reading. That can wait for another time.

Preparation

"Lie down on your back. Do not move. Your stomach expands and contracts slowly like a little balloon. Let your feet, legs, hands, arms grow heavy. Smile a bit while gently closing your eyes. Now we shall travel on a magic carpet to a faraway land."

Relaxation

"You walk on the bank of the river. You hear the monkeys laughing in the trees. The pink flamingo glides noiselessly in the sky. It is hot: go near the waterfall for a sip of fresh water. Everywhere around you there are huge trees, creepers, fragrant flowers of all colours and little cherries that melt in the mouth. The red sun descends on the horizon. It is cooler. The hippopotamus is fast asleep. Soon it shall be the African night. It's time to return."

Waking up

"Breathe deep. Now move your fingers, then the toes. Stretch yourself. Yawn if you wish to. Gently, turn to the side so that you can sit." Without insisting, coax the child to speak about what he felt.

Rounding off

"Stand up. With hands joined in front of the heart, greet yourself while closing your eyes and bowing your head."

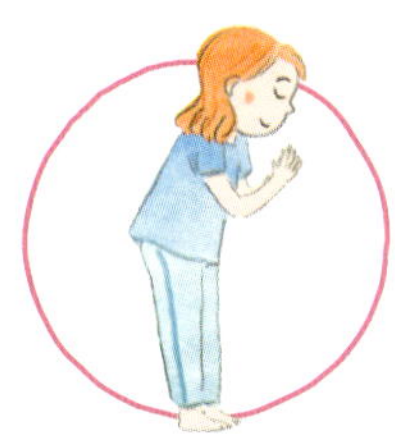

Postures

In the tale, the little monkey looks for ways to please himself: making a nice meal; having fun with his friends; getting the better of those stronger than himself; admiring the beauty of nature... To be able to do all this, he comes across as clever, persevering, wise...without ever losing his cheerful mood! While doing the postures associated with the story, thanks to his body, the child identifies with the happy adventures of Malisco. Therefore, he experiences a positive attitude with which he can realise his desires.
The postures in this book have been taken from classic Indian postures. These have been adapted to the tale and for children.

Opening oneself up to joy

p. 2

Karana

Benefit: Being in an inner state of joy.

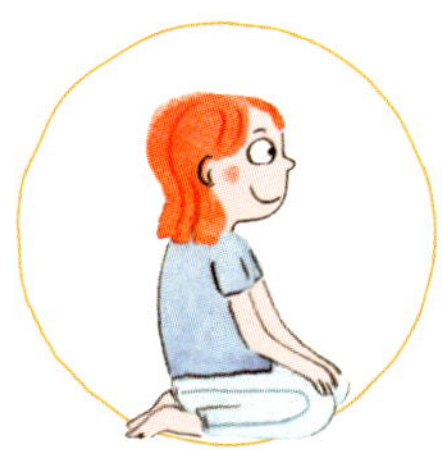

Sit down on your heels and place your hands on your thighs.

4 breaths

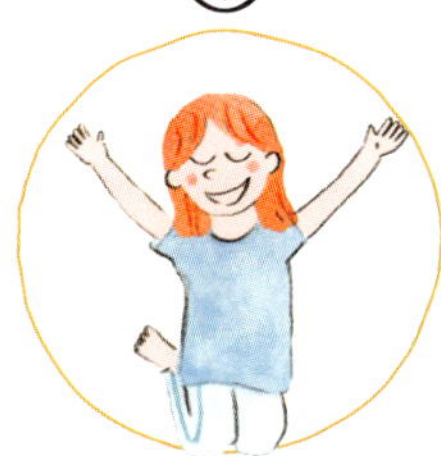

Open your hands, chest, and the palms of your hands wide.

4 breaths

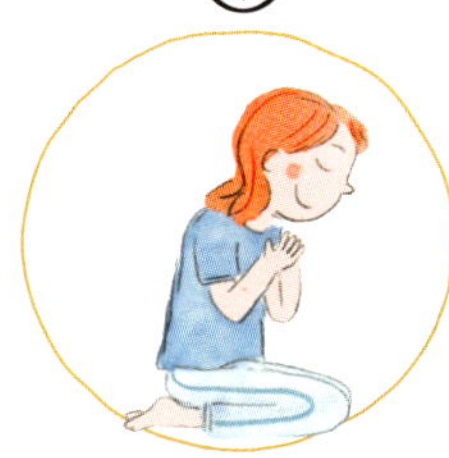

Join your hands in front of your heart and bow your head.

The crocodile

p. 4

Makarasana

Benefit: Toning up the back and shoulder muscles.

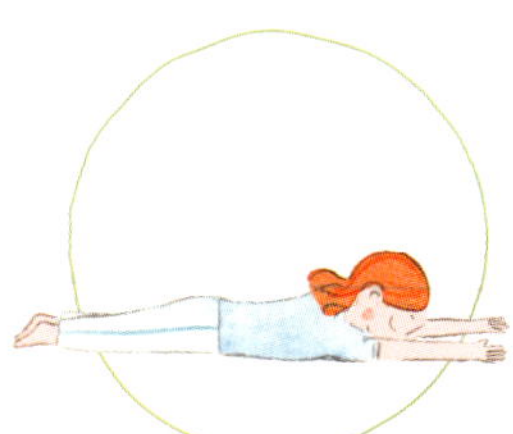

Lie down on your stomach with your hands in front of you.

3 times

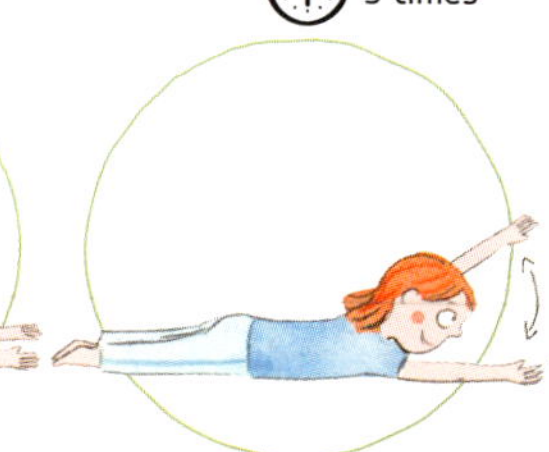

Lift and bring down one of the outstretched hands. Open and close Denduratou's jaws.

3 times

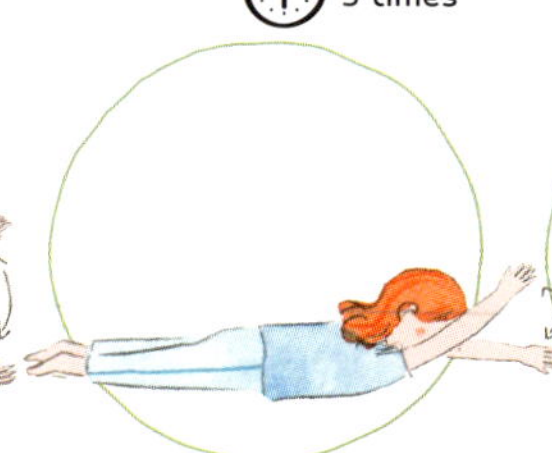

Do the same thing with the other hand.

4 breaths

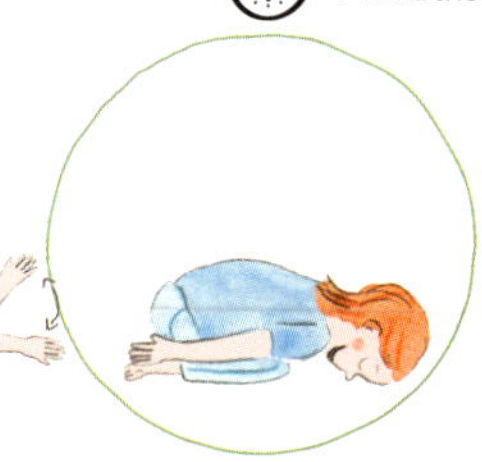

Sit down on your heels and touch the forehead to the ground.

The flight of the pink flamingo
p. 6

Shuttamurgasana

Benefit: Association of balance and movement.

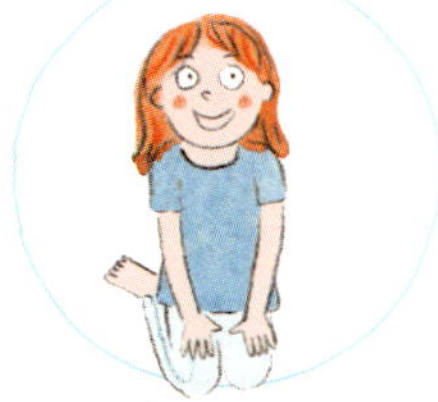

Get down on your knees and sit on your heels.

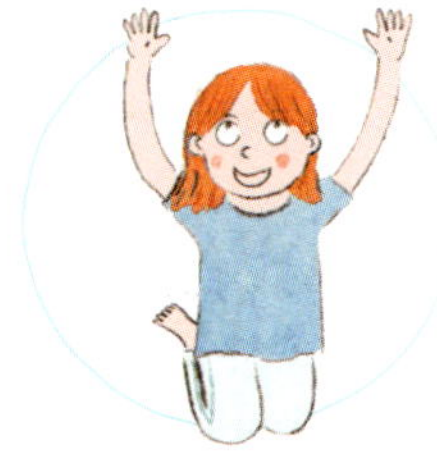

Spread your hands and lift them to the sky.

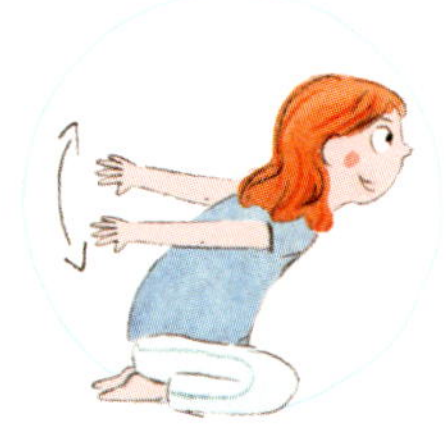

Lean in front and stretch your hands backwards, moving them from the bottom to the top.

4 breaths

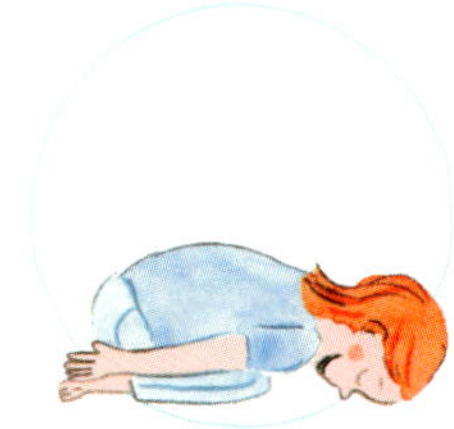

Touch your forehead to the ground, with your hands towards the back.

The elephant and antelope steps
p. 8

Heavy and light.

Benefit: Developing the ability to adapt.

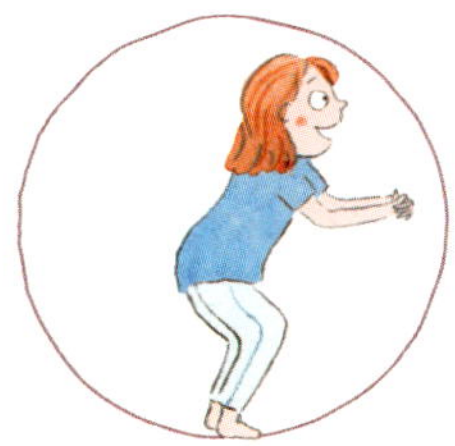

Fold the knees and hold your hands in front of you while crossing the fingers. You are now a trunk!

4 breaths

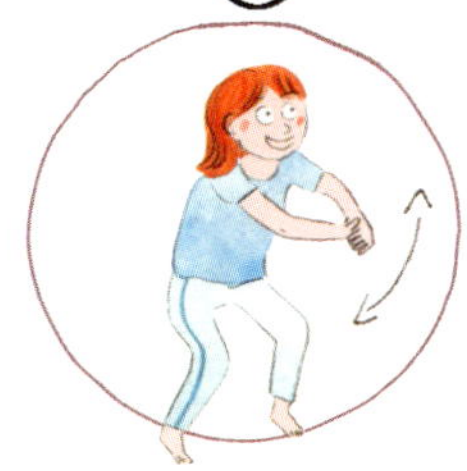

Walk with a heavy step, with your feet apart. Sway your arms from the top to the bottom.

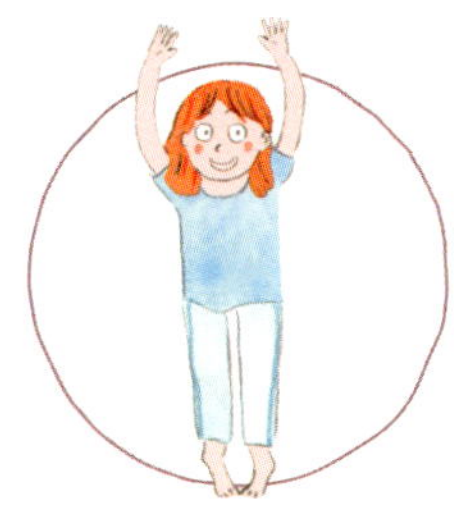

Stand straight on tiptoe and lift your hands.

3 breaths

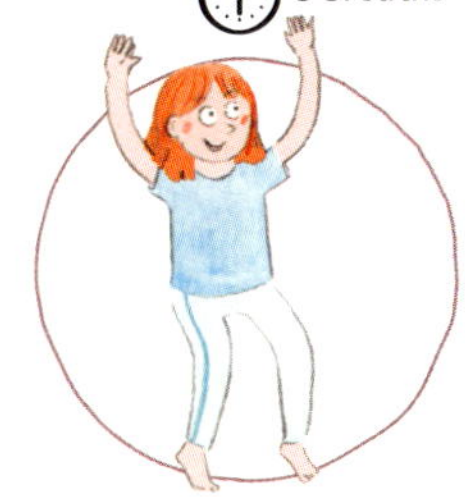

Walk on tiptoe while taking light steps.

Denduratou's tears
p. 14

Pranayama or sobbing breath

Benefit: Regaining energy.

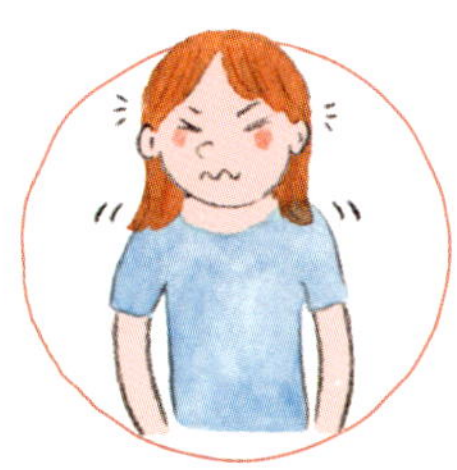

Take many short breaths while inflating the chest as though you were crying!

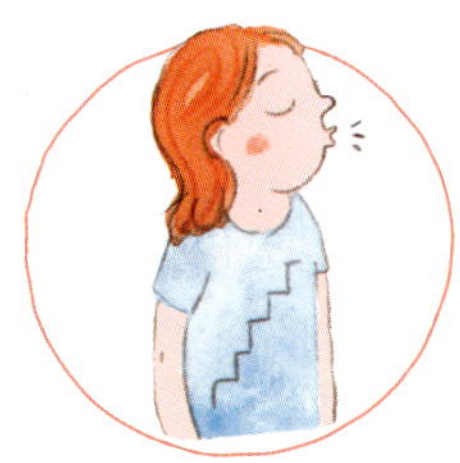

Imagine your breath is climbing stairs.

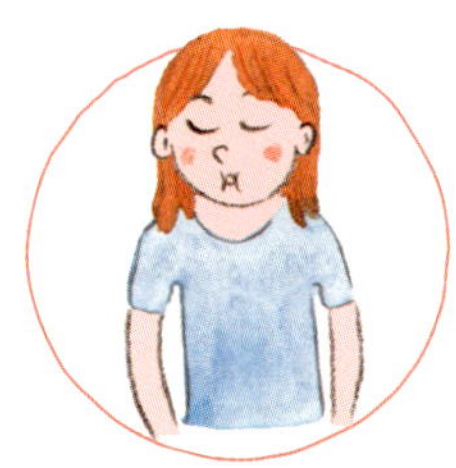

Let out a deep sigh. Repeat all the steps two times.

Carrying coconuts
p. 19

Katasana or the little chair

Benefits: Improvement of the head's position in maintaining balance while walking.

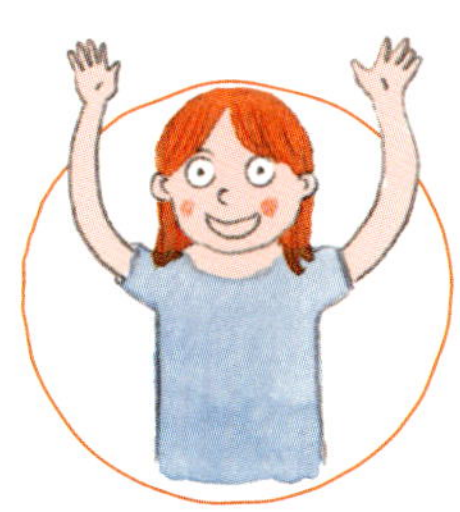

While standing, lift your hands and spread your fingers.

4 breaths

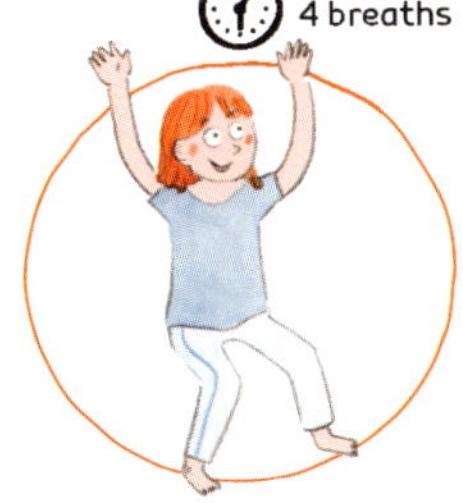

Fold your legs and walk like a monkey.

3 breaths

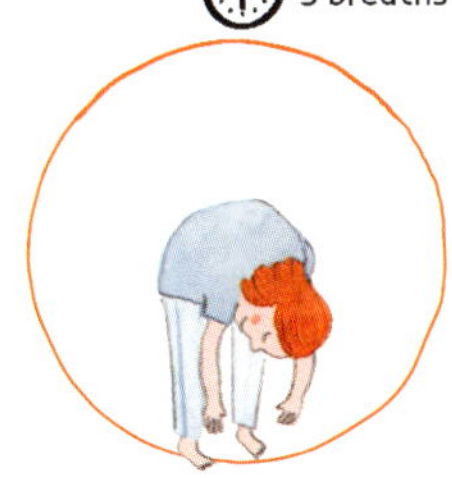

Lean in front, with your legs stretched.

The snake

p. 21

Bhujangasana or the cobra

Benefit: Strengthening the hands and the lower body.

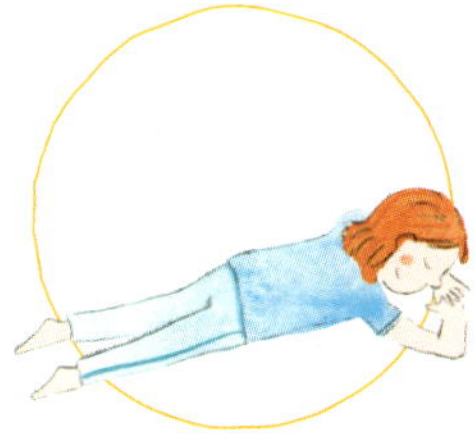

Lie down on the ground and place your forehead on your hands that are on top of each other.

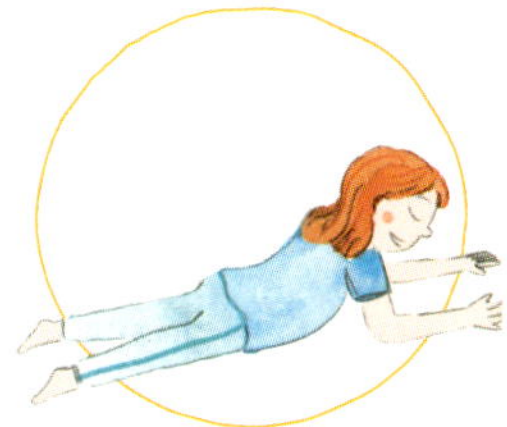

With the help of your elbows, straighten your bust, with your stomach on the ground.

3 breaths

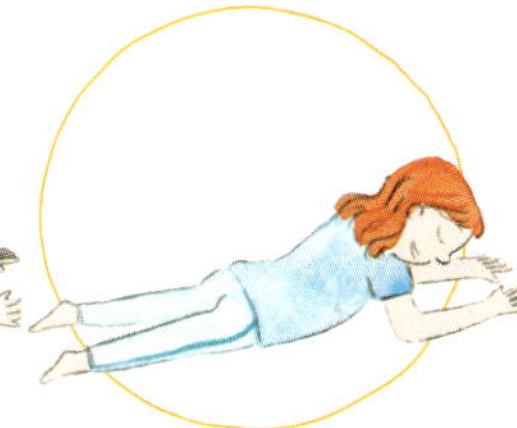

Bring your chin towards your throat.

4 breaths

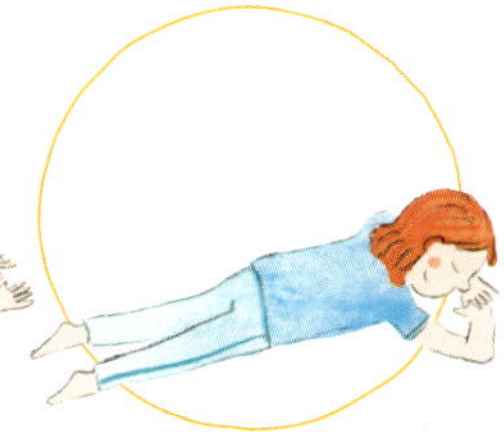

Get back to the original position.

The sail

p. 22

Halasana or the plough (variation)

Benefit: Stretches the spine.

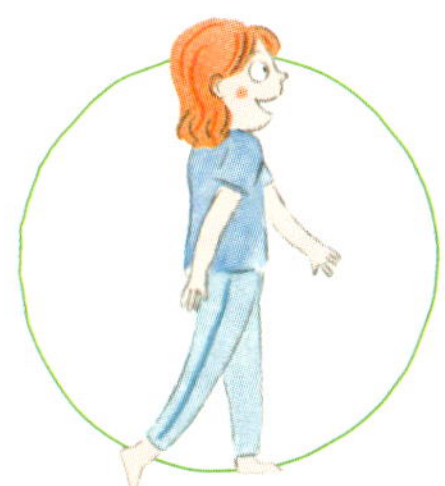

Glide one leg towards the back with the tip of the foot.

3 respirations

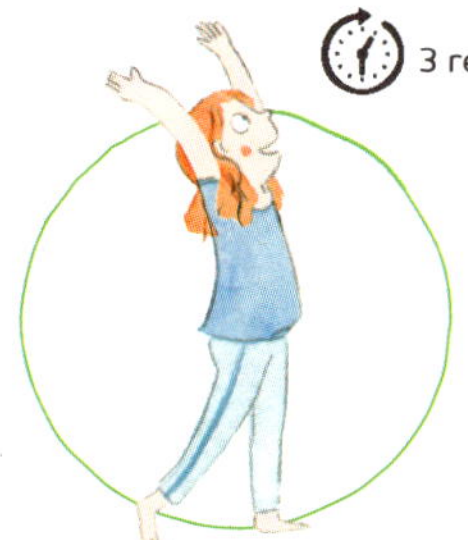

Lift your hands high and a bit towards the back. Thrust out your pelvis.

4 respirations

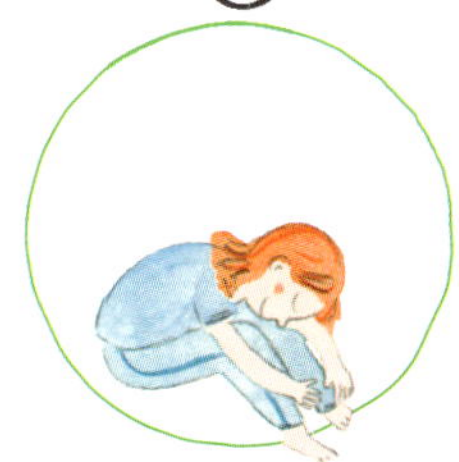

Sit down, fold your legs and place your head on your folded knees.

Crying while laughing

p. 27

Pranayama or the descending breath

Benefit: Good for peace and calm.

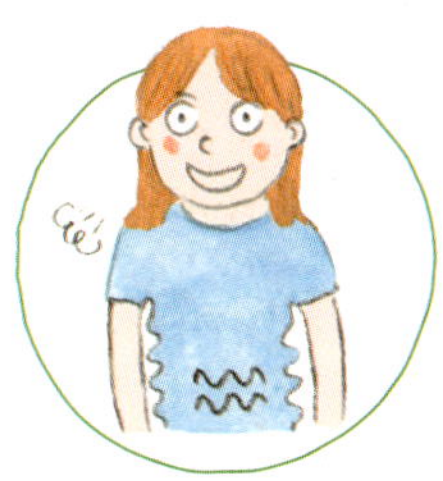

Exhale while shaking your stomach as though you are dying to laugh. The air coming out of your nose makes a noise.

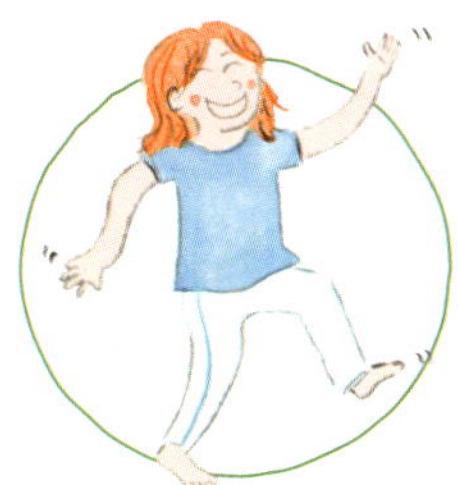

Laugh and dance!